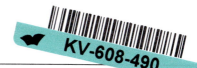

Ethical Dilemmas *in* Healthcare

A PRACTICAL APPROACH THROUGH MEDICAL HUMANITIES

Dr Rowena Murray

Senior Lecturer, Centre for Academic Practice, University of Strathclyde, UK

CHAPMAN & HALL

London · Weinheim · New York · Tokyo · Melbourne · Madras

Published by Chapman & Hall, 2–6 Boundary Row, London SE1 8HN, UK

Chapman & Hall, 2–6 Boundary Row, London SE1 8HN, UK

Chapman & Hall GmbH, Pappelallee 3, 69469 Weinheim, Germany

Chapman & Hall USA, 115 Fifth Avenue, New York NY 10003, USA

Chapman & Hall Japan, ITP-Japan, Kyowa Building, 3F, 2-2-1 Hirakawacho, Chiyoda-ku, Tokyo 102, Japan

Chapman & Hall Australia, 102 Dodds Street, South Melbourne, Victoria 3205, Australia

Chapman & Hall India, R. Seshadri, 32 Second Main Road, CIT East, Madras 600 035, India

Distributed in the USA and Canada by Singular Publishing Group Inc., 4284 41st Street, San Diego, California 92105

First edition 1997

© 1997 Rowena Murray

Typeset in Great Britain by Saxon Graphics Ltd, Derby

Printed in Great Britain by Page Bros, Norwich

ISBN 0 412 62430 3   1 56593 441 5 (USA)

A catalogue record for this book is available from the British Library

Library of Congress Catalog Card Number: 96–86427

♾ Printed on permanent acid-free text paper, manufactured in accordance with ANSI/NISO Z39.48-1992 and ANSI/NISO Z39.48-1984 (Permanence of Paper).

Ethical Dilemmas in Healthcare

'S ON THE INTERNET VIA WWW, GOPHER, FTP OR EMAIL:

WWW:	http://www.thomson.com
GOPHER:	gopher.thomson.com
FTP:	ftp.thomson.com
EMAIL:	findit@kiosk.thomson.com

A service of I(T)P®

For Morag K. Thow

Contents

Preface

This book describes a thought provoking method for exploring issues in healthcare, using literary texts on medical subjects to stimulate discussion. Medical humanities usually prompts a mixture of personal and professional reflections. Above all, it can reveal our patterns of interpretation, our habits of thought and our deep-seated values and assumptions.

A wide range of people have enjoyed this approach (including non-medical people). This book is primarily aimed at health professionals and others who are interested in exploring personal and professional issues in healthcare. Those who are interested in reflective practice can use medical humanities to create 'reflective moments', so that the skills of reflection can be developed. Those who teach undergraduates can use medical humanities for clinical briefing and debriefing, so that students can connect what they hear in the clinic and the classroom and can begin to work through some of the new experiences that clinical placements bring. There may also be an opportunity to develop communication and group work skills. Those who teach postgraduates, in Clinical Reasoning modules, for example, may find medical humanities useful for exploring this topic further. Finally, anyone looking for an excuse to read literature again – this is relevant to our work – will enjoy the extracts and summaries of discussions.

This book is divided into two Parts. Part One gives a general introduction to medical humanities, with definitions, an overview of approaches and texts and reactions from participants. Part Two is a detailed discussion of specific texts which have been used in medical humanities discussions and proved effective in stimulating discussion on a wide range of topics.

The overall aim is to support those who wish to try out this approach for themselves. Details on setting up and managing a medical humanities group are included. Examples of literary texts are included. Even the first advertisement we used for the first meeting of the Glasgow Medical Humanities Group is provided as an exemplar. This book can, therefore, work as a text for other groups. It can also complement the scientific textbook, just as medical humanities can complement the purely medical model of care.

Acknowledgements

In the beginning, I was inspired, by a medic, to use medical humanities as an excuse to get back to literature. I then found that medical humanities could be a way of making 'reflective practice' happen, helping students to engage with complex issues in health care. But in the Glasgow group we have evolved a form of staff development, for medical and non-medical people alike. I learned this from members of the group. These people have captivated me and, I think, each other with their openness, courage and humour in facing up to some tough texts and some nasty probing questions from the group facilitator: me.

Julie Lang, Karen Hughes, Marie Donaghy, Phyllis Campbell and Lynne Pearce read drafts of chapters; your positive feedback was all I needed to write more.

Morag Thow, co-founder of the Glasgow group, brought her professionalism and knowledge to our discussions about this book, while supplying precious reminders of the 'things that matter'.

I am also grateful to the publishers and authors who agreed to let me include extracts of their work: Faber and Faber and Douglas Dunn for the poem 'Second Opinion', from *Elegies*, Macmillan and Elizabeth Jennings for the poem 'After an Operation', from *Collected Poems*, and John Murray for George Mackay Brown's poem 'The Door of Water', from *Winterfold* (with thanks also to Archie Bevan, George Mackay Brown's literary executor). I hope these authors enjoy seeing their work in this new context and I am sorry that GMB did not live to see this book in print, since he was one of the inspirational forces behind it.

Neil MacLennon took the photographs of the Glasgow group.

Part One : GENERAL INTRODUCTION TO MEDICAL HUMANITIES

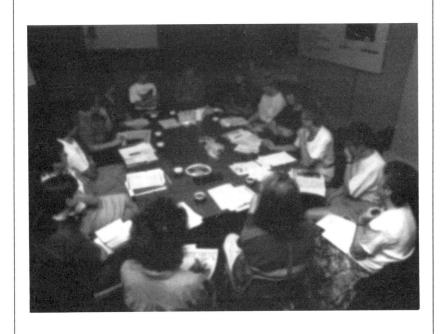

1 Introduction

What is medical humanities? ● *The Glasgow group* ● *Why are you reading this book?* ● *Reactions* ● *Summary: reasons for reading*

What is medical humanities?

Literature and medicine

Medical humanities, as I know it, simply means using literature in a medical discussion. In parallel with the usual textbook, a literary text can encourage us to explore difficult issues or simply to work out our own views. We can use literary texts to stimulate discussion of health care. The free-wheeling discussion that a literary text can provoke draws out both personal and professional views.

In medical humanities we use literary texts to stimulate discussion, with the aim of not excluding personal views and personal interpretation. The point is to bring this personal dimension back into discussions of 'medical' topics. It is this personal dimension that makes people make time for the discussions.

Free reflection

A dynamic discussion of a poem on a medical topic can provoke expressions of both professional and personal views.

This mix can be very stimulating, not only for individuals who may only have been able to express complaints about constraints in health care in informal discussion, but also for the whole group, which can become a forum for free reflection. If the group is managed well, there are no sanctions against mixing personal and professional reflection. Are we given this freedom anywhere else in our professional lives?

Safe forum

This kind of forum is, I would argue, unique. Over time it can allow individuals, both medical and non-medical, not only to express views but also to develop them.

For example, we all have our own views on genetic engineering, but how often do we discuss this topic, reflect on and review our assumptions? There are questions which we need to revisit from time to time, such as: Is it 'right' to progress with scientific discovery first and resolve ethical dilemmas second? Do you think that individual cases must be judged on their own merits? Do you think the end justifies the means, or not? Do you think that the rights and wrongs depend on beliefs about the beginning of life, about when life can be said to have begun? Does this view then shape your judgements of the scientific advances and prospects? And is the issue further complicated by age, gender, race or colour of the patients or the health professionals, or not, in your view?

Furthermore, if we do discuss this topic, how often do we have the chance to listen to others' views, to interact with them, to question them, to change our minds, or not, or to focus our thinking, without being driven and directed by aims and assessments or 'authorities' and 'superiors'? How often do we have this kind of safe forum?

Genetic engineering is one of the big issues of our time, but there are also the equally demanding – perhaps more demanding – smaller issues, the daily dilemmas. For example, there is the dilemma of how much, or how little, time to spend with a patient or with a patient's relative. There is also the gap between the 'real' and the 'ideal' in professional practice, where we have to compromise with the prevailing culture of the ward, the Trust or the government. There may even be a gap between health professionals, which can create a daily struggle to make yourself heard across the hierarchical divide. Such daily dilemmas may be just as difficult to resolve. They may be very wearying and undermining of our health and confidence, particularly if they stay unexamined and unresolved.

Literary texts: open to interpretation

'Literature' can be intimidating to some people, but then so can 'medical' subjects. Talking about either subject takes some skill and confidence, especially if we include in that talk, for once, our personal views, our opinions and even our deeply embedded assumptions.

The literary text itself opens up issues, since it is open to more than one interpretation. This openness is new to many people who have not continued to read literature in their professional years and to students of science, among others, who may rarely or never have participated in a literary discussion. In medical humanities we exploit this openness in the text to enable discussion of different sides of the issues. For example, it is difficult to maintain the 'diagnosis → treatment' pattern of thought once a group of health professionals has produced widely differing interpretations of the medical subject. This is further complicated by the mixture of the personal and the professional in these interpretations. The medical subject quickly becomes more diffuse, more complex, more ambivalent and the discussion becomes richer, more flexible, more creative and more 'playful'.

Many literary discussions would begin by concentrating on a number of 'legitimate' interpretations of a text that could be made without background information, and a medical humanities discussion will also focus on the text in this way, while participants are encouraged to locate their interpretations in the words in front of them. Each reader can be enabled to make an interpretation, even if only of one or two lines that have caught their attention, through a combination of individual (private) writing and discussion in pairs, before a plenary discussion involving the whole group.

Medical experience: narration and reflection

After this initial engagement with the text, participants usually draw on their own experience and often incorporate it into their interpretation of the poem. This is where participants can negotiate the distinctions and overlaps between their own readings, other people's readings and their own assumptions and expectations.

It is the medical subject of the poem, short story, novel or dramatic extract that works as a prompt for a group of health professionals (and people who have been or seen patients), giving them something to get their teeth into. It is familiar ground. People usually narrate from their experiences as health professionals, patients or carers, telling stories of experiences related to those in the literary text they have just read.

But we also have to engage with what the text actually says. It will inevitably have some features, particular to context or character, individual or institution, which do not match our own experience. This can encourage us to reflect not only on our experience but also on our patterns of interpretation. This is one of the healthy side-effects of medical humanities.

Personal and professional development

Medical humanities provides a unique forum for continuing professional and personal development. Topics that are not covered after graduation may stagnate if there is no opportunity for reflection and development.

For example, issues of personal beliefs, health-care philosophies, attitudes to health policies, clinical reasoning skills and differences in professional practice, which might have been quite thoroughly dealt with in the undergraduate years, may never be dealt with again. This is a heavy burden for the individual – to develop these aspects without structure and support.

Sometimes a medical humanities discussion leads to a sudden realization of a very specific aspect of our professional practice which needs to be changed. However, it is not possible to know precisely what people take from discussions, since we have no 'accounting', no totalling up of ground covered, or shifted, by each individual by the end of each discussion. This is not possible if the writing and small-group work are private. What I have observed is that people enjoy alternating between narration and reflection in this way.

What are the outcomes? How do you know it works?

Perhaps I should pause here. There is a risk of appearing to claim too much for medical humanities – more than I can document at this time.

However, this introduction is based not only on my own observations, but also on participants' reactions in the Glasgow medical humanities group over the past 5 years, in discussions with students and patients and in conference presentations and other one-off workshops.

The effect of this technique, either in one-off sessions or longer-term has not been measured in any scientific way. In fact, a recent article, written by members of one of the first medical humanities departments in a medical faculty, at Pennsylvania State University, highlights this question of the impact of this approach as the focus for future research. In the meantime, comments from regular participants in a medical humanities group are included to give an impression of the impact of what seems to current practitioners to be a technique that has immense value.

Dialogue

It is not always easy to say what you think. If there is debate and dispute about a point, if, in fact, it is inherently debatable, this can be demanding, even stressful.

The discussion can be genuinely wide-ranging enough to challenge our views. If people deal with each other, and themselves, with patience and respect, if they care for each other when the issue is troubling, then we can deal with difficult issues, with the difficulty of difference and with potentially destructive voices or issues in others or in ourselves.

Perhaps the skills of articulating a view, be it an ideal or a disagreement, or of simply stating your own view, are best maintained by practice.

Fun

There is one final point that must be stressed: participants enjoy medical humanities.

All of these groups have reported that they enjoy medical humanities. The Glasgow group meets every 6–8 weeks, for 2½ hours, in the evening. Some people have attended all the meetings over 5 years; others drift in and out, depending on other commitments. They give up their time for no tangible professional gain. Would they do this if they did not enjoy it?

The Glasgow group

My first contact with medical humanities was in January 1991, through a medic who was a fellow participant in 'Teaching and Learning in Higher Education', an academic staff development course. During one of the breaks, when all the good discussion goes on, we began to talk about what makes people learn best. The talk turned to medical education and he did not mince his words: it was his view that medicine attracts people who want to care for others, but that medical education soon grinds that out of them, leaving some 'scarred for life'. Medical education, for him, had been a programme of rote learning and socialization into an elite.

Whether or not you or I agree with this version of medical education, we can recognize in his story that sense of constraint on both learners and practitioners who try to practise both the art and science of caring and curing.

He then started to talk about this approach called 'medical humanities' and later sent me two papers on the subject. These gave me not only a clear definition of the approach but also examples of literature that had been used in medical education in the USA.

I am not a medic. All I know about medical education is based on reading and talking to people who have studied medicine, nursing or physiotherapy. My background is in literature. To me, medical humanities seemed an effective way to make literature useful and accessible to a wider audience. People could talk about poems not just for the sake of interpreting them, or for teaching and publishing their interpretations, but in order to develop their skills and to communicate better with each other. Above all, literature could provide the art and artistry to complement a heavy scientific bias.

While this might sound to literary purists like a degradation of the grand designs and lofty purposes of literature, I felt I had stumbled on a way to make literature less exclusive. Literary specialists could always talk about literature; now others could be included, could generate their own discussions.

An enthusiastic physiotherapist called Morag Thow took the imaginative leap of suggesting that we set up our own medical humanities group: she brought the people and I brought the poems and questions. We publicized the event on a very simple poster at hospitals, colleges and universities in the area. A small group turned up at the first evening, intrigued by the innovative idea and/or persuaded along by one of us.

Since then the group, of between 10 and 15 at any meeting, has become a regular event, attracting nurses, physiotherapists, secretaries, educators, clinicians, midwives, librarians, students and teachers of other subjects and other non-medical people. There is no fixed group identity; people turn up when they can and new people come along from time to time, bringing new perspectives, new questions and new responses. Perhaps this mix is one of the most important features of our group.

We use poems, short stories and extracts from novels, and I add newspaper or journal articles to bring out different angles on topics such as HRT, mental health, disability, the elderly and the ageing population, genetic engineering, cancer, etc. Often our discussions return to the processes of power and institutionalization, from the points of view of carers and patients. We have gathered together a wide range of texts, covering diverse themes, including topical issues as they come up in the media. This book offers a selection of these texts, providing texts, questions and prompts for discussion, with extracts from actual discussions.

Our skills in textual analysis have developed over time, along with the confidence not to reject a poem that proves difficult but to take time over it.

Group work is a growth area in education and I wanted to develop my own skills, and the skills of the other group members, in this area. In my role at the Centre for Academic Practice (Strathclyde University) I have a staff development responsibility and I have been looking at techniques for working with academic staff, both experienced and inexperienced. My research on reflective practice among academic staff at Strathclyde suggests that this kind of safe forum for discussion of innovation is essential for sustained and effective professional development.

Collaborative papers, conference presentations and a Medical Humanities Roadshow (sponsored by Ferrier's Medical Booksellers, Edinburgh) have helped me to develop my ideas. For example, at the World Congress for Physical Therapy in 1995 my presentation, co-authored with Morag Thow, focused on the need to develop the human, not just clinical, skills which are covered in undergraduate years but often neglected after graduation. This proposition was warmly received by the international group who attended and medical humanities was seen to be an effective way of developing a range of skills appropriate for health professionals. If the feedback from this, as from other presentations, is so good then there must be a place for medical humanities in the education of health professionals. The question of whether this should be during undergraduate study or after is still open.

I am writing this textbook in the hope that it will 'spread the word' beyond the successful Glasgow group. I hope that people will adopt or adapt my material and run their own groups, or try out this technique with undergraduates (hence the 'how to' approach of later chapters). I would also be happy if it stimulated one or two people to take up reading literature again.

Why are you reading this book?

Does this idea of running your own group seem far-fetched? You feel you do not know enough about literature to handle, let alone lead, a discussion about a poem? Chapter 2 tells you exactly what to do. Chapter 5 gives you one of the first examples I used, the poem 'After an Operation' by Elizabeth Jennings. We also used this poem on the roadshow and found that people took to the discussion very quickly. It has proved itself as a good place to start.

This book could, then, be used as a course text, with the literary texts complementing the scientific texts. I prefer the process of adding literary texts throughout a course to isolating them to a discrete module, because this might achieve better integration of the art and science in the learning and practice.

People who might be interested in this book could be identified by their profession, i.e. any profession with a medical/health role. Yet non-medical people have joined our group and made an important contribution to the discussions (myself included!). In fact, you may well have picked up this book because it is **not** related to your profession, not in the usual, scientific way at least. This personal interest is, I think, what keeps people coming back to our medical humanities group; i.e. there is room in the kind of discussion we have for a wide range of interests, motives and development.

Reactions

That people have come to the group with a variety of agendas and interests is evident from these extracts from answers to a semi-structured questionnaire. Here are some of the questions, with representative extracts from participants' answers:

What did you think of 'literature' before you first came to this group?

Before coming to the group I thought of literature as of source of pleasure, an indulgence. Poetry has always made me feel relaxed. Authors like Gerald Durrell and G. M. Fraser make me laugh and lighten my mood. So I have always selected literature as a means of enhancing or changing a mood state. I have loved books and reading for as long as I can remember. However, now I read so many textbooks and journal articles to enhance my teaching material that the time to read for pleasure is restricted. I feel sad about this and particularly about not having the time to **browse** through lots of books.

I sometimes think that some of the pieces we discuss go 'over the top'. This kind of writing seems to me to be 'in vogue' just now along with all the interest in alternative medicine and medic bashing. At least the discussions may 'go over the top'. I agree if people have a grievance or have had a bad experience they feel the need to share with others, well and good, but a lot of people jump on the bandwagon so to speak and a lot of rubbish is written.

Literature sounded very 'highbrow'. Have read very little literature until now. Knew it was useful but didn't seem to have time to read any.

I find I don't have time to read the things I would like to as most reading for pleasure time I have is short and I just want a quick 'fix' of words and story and don't have the self-discipline to analyse what I am reading. I feel reading literature is essential to a person whose work involves communication with people of varying vocabulary and intellect in order to communicate effectively.

Have you changed any of these views since then?

Yes the group has shifted my perspective of literature. I can see literary works can be a useful tool to stimulate discussion, raise issues, gain insight into personal experiences that can be used as a focus for thoughts with students. This way I can read for plea- sure and for work and not feel guilty.

The group gives me a structure, where time has been set aside to read and think.

Working with the group has helped me to look more closely at the extracts and articles and to discuss their relevance to health issues. I feel it will encourage me to read more widely, expanding the strictly medical approach. My definition of 'literature' is much the same. I have seen how it can throw light on difficult moral or ethical problems.

Enjoyed most of the literature used. Have started to build up books on literature and beginning to read more widely.

Have your group work skills developed as a result of working in this group?

I probably have learned to listen more and have realized I often speak too soon before really considering properly. I don't have much experience of group work but in my working life I certain- ly try to listen properly to my 'patients'/'clients' and do my best to help them and while not a proper counsellor I have been on a counselling course now because of my interest. I seem to have had some success.

No! I still talk too much but that's because I find the group excit- ing and have difficulty containing my enthusiasm.

Has your attitude to writing – i.e. doing some writing – changed as a result of working in this group?

Not really.... There always seems so much to do in the evening after work and I have other preferred activities and I think maybe I'm lazy as I would always opt for reading rather than writing. It takes me all my time to keep up my correspondence with friends abroad! A much less threatening role. Where before I was more con- cerned about my quality, this is safe and I can express freely.

Has being in the group affected how you teach and/or how you do your job?

Yes.... I think I am able to understand the students better than perhaps some other staff. I can usually sense when people are unhappy or 'not themselves'. I try to help the students adopt a more holistic approach to their patients and listen to what **they** would like the outcome to be rather than what the physio thinks – in other words we try to come to mutual short- and long-term aims or goals with reviews of progress.

I feel more supported in my own way of working with patients and my interest in their experience of hospital/being unwell/body image change/medical staff. I have discussed Medical Humanities issues in staff room and pinned up interesting and relevant info on the noticeboard and many staff have also read the May Sarton ('After the Stroke') and 'Body Silent' (Murphy) – so it has heightened their awareness of the patient and their feelings and experience also.

Yes – using more literature and patients' views on illness and health in my teaching. Students beginning to explore the arts, etc.

Not so far, but I can see ways in which it might.

Comments from participants, even in one-off sessions, show that initial fears of literature, Literature with a capital L, can be overcome. In fact, the fear of literature could be a good talking point in itself.

Health professionals have been enabled to trust their own impressions and to shape and share their own interpretations. They have been instructed in the skills of analysis. They have practised articulating their views in short, informal, private writings. They now continue to develop their skills.

A safety net has helped: ground rules and good facilitation have helped in heated debate and disagreement. Complex issues have naturally produced a wide range of views. There has been no drive towards a consensus. Nor have we worked for 'professional outcomes', which might connect our discussion with the workplace. Yet some of the reposes show that there is an effect on professional practice. This apparent lack of direction has helped us to keep our discussions genuinely open-ended.

Is this, therefore, relevant to the health professional's workplace? For some there is an instant effect – for example, the nurse who, after reading Elizabeth Jennings's poem 'After an Operation' realized that she had forgotten to tell a patient how she would feel when she woke up. Others have enjoyed reading for its own sake. Some see the effect as purely personal; they feel medical humanities is something they do for themselves.

For students medical humanities has had a similar effect, though timing can affect their responses. For example, as they prepare for their first clinical experience they can begin, through the study of literature, to think about contexts for health care. Perhaps more importantly, they can begin to think about their own assumptions and values. They can also keep in touch with the human side of care and the patient's point of view, thus complementing the purely medical model of care. Unlike a medical case study, where the activity often becomes a process of finding the right answer, the literary 'case' may have no right or wrong answers; the work is all in **interpretation**. The period after clinical experience would seem to be another opportunity to use literature to tease out reflections on new experiences, conflicts, difficult issues and daily dilemmas, in a form of 'clinical debriefing'.

Summary: reasons for reading

- For fun. Read some literature. Follow the discussions. Wonder about the point of it all later, or not at all. Enjoy not reading for work.
- For work. You can build this material into a course. A medical humanities text – for example, a poem like 'After an Operation' – can complement the clinical textbook.
- For yourself. You can get together a group of friends or colleagues, or both, to compare reactions, to revive the human side of caring, to explore professional and personal dilemmas in health care.
- For writing. Do some scribbling, in any form, on any topic, for no more than 10 minutes. Enjoy private writing. Enjoy saying what you really think.
- For research: the benefits of medical humanities are clear to its experienced practitioners but as yet there has been hardly any work in evaluating it, in analysing its effects, in studying these scientifically.
- Not to become a more caring person – this is not the goal, although it may be one of the side-effects.

2 How to run a medical humanities group

Step-by-step guide ● Managing the debate ● Guidelines on patterns of discussion ● Techniques for focusing on the text ● Complementary texts: scientific and literary ● Complementary discussion: narration and reflection ● Complementary outcomes: personal and professional observations

---

Step-by-step guide

Readers who have experience in running groups might want to skip this section, although it might still have some use in showing how to apply existing skills in this new context.

To start: there need be no fixed agenda for a medical humanities session. Instead, there are focal points in the literary text that prompt different interpretations, and individual beliefs and experiences that can shape those interpretations. A short poem is a good starting point. There are no stated aims and objectives, but perhaps there needs to be a general shared purpose, particularly for the first meeting: for example, 'to try out a new approach called Medical Humanities', or 'to explore a difficult topic, like patient-centred care or genetic engineering', or 'it's an excuse for reading literature again' and 'it will be enjoyable and stimulating'. People will need a reason for turning up. If coffee and tea are provided, so much the better.

Our advertisement for our first session included an open invitation, a brief definition, a couple of examples, along with details of time, venue and contact names. Figure 2.1 shows exactly how it looked.

There is no formal or informal assessment, although people can and probably should be invited to say what they think about this new approach. A medical humanities group can therefore be independent from other professional structures. Moreover, everyone can have a say in how it develops.

Medical humanities
A Discussion Group
for
Physiotherapists, nurses, doctors, etc.

What?   What can the 'humanities' – literature, philosophy, etc. – tell us about medical care? Novels, short stories and poems can provide provocative insights and starting points for discussions of different views. For example, May Sarton's *After the Stroke* gives the patient's view of illness and treatments. Solzhenitsyn's *Cancer Ward* is another example of a work of literature which focuses on the medical world.
In this discussion group we will read extracts from works of literature and consider different experiences of health care, different medical conditions and their treatments and different views of the medical world.

When?   Thursdays 7–9 pm
Starting 28 June, 1990

Where?   Gartnavel General Hospital

Who?   Morag Thow   Tel XXX XXX XXXX
Rowena Murray Tel XXX XXX XXXX ext XXXX

No enrolment necessary

Figure 2.1 Original advertisement used by the Glasgow group.

All of the above needs to be aired in an initial briefing at the first meeting. Any member of the group can take responsibility for doing this (although it has been our choice to keep one person in the role of chair throughout 5 years). This person also has to undertake to encourage and support participants as they attempt to read and respond to poetry, for example, for what may be the first time in many years. In addition, the writing exercises, which aim to help people develop a view, may at first be daunting; i.e. being asked to **do** writing. In fact, almost everyone in our group has enjoyed writing **for themselves**.

Is a literary specialist needed? It helps if there is someone with techniques in literary analysis in their background. Literary skills are useful in unpacking literary texts and in teaching others how to do so. However, working with examples in this text should help readers to develop the basic skills. There are frameworks here for six sessions, including general guidelines on dealing with literary texts and hints on managing the discussion of a specific text.

Above all, whoever chairs the discussions must avoid becoming the 'filter' for the discussion or the dominant expert (even if they are the most expert on a particular topic). The aim is not to get at the 'right' interpretation but to include a wide range of views, as wide a range as is represented in the group, whether they be experts or not.

Since running a group discussion without a fixed agenda, preserving this kind of openness, is a challenge, it might be useful to consider what has emerged as the general pattern of discussion in our medical humanities group. Intended as a framework for new groups, here is a streamlined, step-by-step guide to chairing a medical humanities session.

Step-by-step guide – 1st meeting: 2 hours

Prepare
1. Select reading(s), find venue, make up poster, spread the word
2. Advertise, distribute poster, lobby contacts
3. Organize coffee, etc.

Facilitate
4. **Welcome**: introductions (10 min)
5. **Briefing**: general purpose, definition of medical humanities, activities, framework for discussions (5 min)
6. **Reactions**: questions, initial reactions (5 min)
7. **Activity**: reading short literary text (5 min)
8. **Activity**: individual private writing (5 min)
9. **Pair-share**: discussion of writings and views (10 min)

Coffee break (15 min)
10. **Groups**: (fours or sixes): compare views (15 min)
11. **Plenary**: whole-group discussion (30 min)
12. **Activity**: writing summary, revise or consolidate view (5 min)
13. **Review of this session** (15 min)
14. Reactions to medical humanities
15. Next meeting: date, venue, chair, admin
16. Materials for next meeting: texts, activities

Managing the debate

The key to starting debate on a literary text seems to me to be to give people time – say, 5 minutes – to write their own views and, crucially, not to ask them to show their writing to anyone else. This gives everyone a starting point, their own 'gut reaction', their own answer to a question posed by the chairperson, or a summary, or whatever they choose to write about. To get people started, 'freewriting', i.e. writing that is continuous, non-stop, without editing, in sentences (not notes) but without structure, always works. I see writing as having an essential role in helping people to develop a view.

Some people prefer to start with a focus; others prefer to have an open remit for their writing. So the writing prompt could be directed and focused or it could be open-ended and unfocused, or both could be offered, allowing people to make their own choice.

Once they have done some writing, a graduated sequence of discussion activities can help debate to develop: starting with 'pair-share' – discussion with one partner; then small-group work – combining pairs in fours or sixes; and finally a whole-group plenary. A final individual private writing activity allows individuals time to take stock of their own views after all this discussion. This sequence of activities can provide a loose structure for both debate and individual reflection. The facilitator can make sure there is variety in the combinations – in pairs, fours and sixes – by asking specific people to work together or by asking the group to mix up the combinations over the weeks.

Confidentiality is a topic on which the facilitator can, and probably should, set some basic ground rules. For example, I asked participants in our first meeting to regard discussions as confidential, unless they had permission from speakers to repeat what they had said outside this discussion. Over time, these ground rules can be revised and agreed by the group. The inclusion of new participants in many sessions probably means that we should revisit this issue from time to time.

The structure of a medical humanities discussion is loose. However, if there are no aims and objectives there is a sharp focus on the text. Discussions can roam widely, including generalizations, personal experiences and medical case histories, but the discussion has to be brought back to the text regularly. Someone has to take responsibility for doing this.

Guidelines on patterns of discussion

Many of our discussions have circled back to issues of power – who has the power to decide? – and institutionalization – how do people lose their power, or autonomy, in a large institution like a hospital? While we strenuously avoid what we have come to call 'medic bashing', we do frequently end up with a critique of the hierarchy of health professionals as itself a source of problems and of barriers to solving them.

While each discussion has a different rhythm and tack there is always an alternating pattern of narration and reflection. People narrate their own experiences, reflect on the experience described in the text, then may take up narration again, with the chairperson bringing the focus back to the text for further reflection, and so on.

There are rarely dead ends. The discussion rarely peters out. This is partly the result of the sequence of individual, pair-share, small-group and whole-group discussions. But it may be stimulating and perhaps reassuring to novices to have more than one text per session and more than one kind of text: combining a poem, a research paper and a newspaper article can open up different sides of the issue and different responses to it, both medical and personal.

Ultimately the medical humanities discussion, even on complex issues like euthanasia, which touches everyone's deepest feelings and deep-seated beliefs about life and medicine, can be highly charged, confusing and yet safe. People give each other respectful and thoughtful attention, since individual viewpoints and expressions come to be expected (though they may still be questioned). Because the poem is not a case study there is no imperative to solve a problem. There is freedom from the task of working towards a common goal in that sense. What people take from the discussion is up to them. That remains private.

There have therefore been recurring issues and repeating patterns in our discussions. A new group could use these questions as points of reflection, to trigger review of the group's work: i.e. will other groups have the same patterns to their discussions?

Techniques for focusing on the text

People drift off the text in discussion in many ways: relating text to their own experience as patients, or to their own practice as health professionals, or to something they have read or heard about. This is important, but it is only part of the medical humanities discussion; the role of the group leader is to balance narration and reflection. Since this 'drifting' is often triggered by the text, the discussion leader can focus on that point in the text. Focusing on a line or two, or on the multiple meanings of one word, in its context, is often all that is needed to return the focus of the discussion to the text:

Questions for focusing discussion on the text

How does that relate to the text?
Do you think that is what is being said in the poem?
Is that the point of view of the person in the text?
How does the word ... relate to what you have just said?

i.e. to prompt individual observations on the text

These questions can be particularly useful throughout the first few meetings of a new group, since participants will not be used to focusing on individual words and opening up layers of meaning in this way. They may reply that the meaning of the word is 'obvious', and therefore need to be encouraged to spell it out. They may assume that everyone will have the same interpretation of a word. (And they may, or may not, be right.)

Sooner or later someone could and probably should ask the question 'Why?': why should we focus on the text? There are many possible answers: asking each member of the group to write down their own answer, and then to compare answers, is an interesting way of moving the discussion on in a way that involves everyone. Similarly, definition exercises, of both simple and complex words, often reveal the diversity of interpretations within the group itself. A follow-up to this can be to consider, individually and then as a group, which definition best suits the context.

One technique for focusing on the text that I have never used is reading it aloud, since I feel that that would begin to put an interpretation on the text. I prefer to leave the reading to the readers in the group.

I do select what I think are key words or phrases in the text before-hand and draw attention to these in discussion. Often I do this simply by asking 'What do you think this means?' – simple questions in simple language, with many variations:

Which words caught your attention, as you were reading?

Why has it been written that way?
Why did the writer choose that word?
How does this line relate to the bit before?
Did anyone else notice this line?
Are there other lines that stand out?

What do you think this means?

There will be focal points in every text, though we may not agree on what they are. In my role as discussion leader I am quite happy if participants focus on any part of the text to the point of analysing, interpreting or responding to it. My techniques for focusing on the text are ultimately aimed at getting everyone in the group to find their own focus and to develop that in discussion.

Examples of these techniques in practice, and in more detail, are given in Chapters 5–10. These chapters include fragments from actual medical humanities conversations and summaries of debates.

Complementary texts: scientific and literary

Undergraduate course work in health studies is science-rich and art-poor. Yet there is an art, or artistry, side to caring. Even artistry can be studied in a scientific mode, i.e. as a set of techniques, another discipline to master. Where the social sciences do appear in the curriculum there may be little integration with science courses. Generally speaking there is a science–arts divide and texts that have more arts than science in them are rarely seen and even more rarely read.

If this is a weakness, then combining literary texts with scientific or medical texts on a specific topic would help, and could bridge the gap. These texts could be 'complementary' in the sense that, taken together, they cover both the art and the science of the subject and could provoke both scientific and personal thinking. Literature has also been used to stimulate discussion among patients; reading a poem, for example, has been used to trigger expression of feelings and thoughts.

It can have the same effect for students, helping them to express a variety of powerful emotions, which might have no other form of release.

For example, the following four texts show different approaches to defining health and disease, in scientific and literary texts:

A few recent or current studies have been looking at physical activity, fitness, and longevity. Professor Jeremy N. Morris of the London School of Hygiene and Tropical Medicine, who together with his colleagues pioneered studies of vigorous exercise and CHD (14, 15), has extended those analyses to all-cause mortality or longevity among British civil servants (12, 13). The first deck of Table 7.1(A) is an excerpt of findings on rates and relative risks of CHD during a 9-year follow-up among 9376 subjects, 45–65 years at entry in 1976, by patterns of sportsplaying characterized by intensity, duration, and frequency.

Paffenbarger, R. S. *et al.* (1994) Some interrelations of physical activity, physiological fitness, health, and longevity, in *Physical Activity, Fitness, and Health: International Proceedings and Consensus Statement*, (eds C. Bouchard *et al.*), Human Kinetics, Windsor, ON, p. 120

Although it has augmented the simplistic binary opposition of health and disease with the parallel notion of illness, the positive and negative aspects of health care are still seen as inversely proportional; i.e. the presence of illness implies a corresponding loss of health.

Sim, J. (1990) The concept of health. *Physiotherapy*, **76**(7), p. 425

Lack of physical and material resources [are] major problems, and it is these things which handicap us, not our disabilities.

Morris, J. (ed.) (1989) *Able Lives*, p. 129

And now I'm convalescent, fear can claim
No general power. Yet I am not the same.
Elizabeth Jennings, 'After an Operation'

The differences between these four texts are more than just stylistic; they each represent a different point of view, they each sit in a different context and each is located within a different value system. Maintaining the 'value' of each type of text, of each point of view and of each person in the health care literature – both scientific and artistic – is frequently a challenge, since each community tends to attach more value to its own texts. This is one of the aims of medical humanities: to show how this variety of texts can produce a richer picture and a richer discussion of health and disease.

Complementary discussion: narration and reflection

People with different backgrounds, or with different education and training, or with different professional roles and responsibilities, may have different responses to medical humanities:

> Importance of shared experience both with the writer and with another person. Access to the unconscious process.
> I try to help the students adopt a more holistic approach to their patients.

These comments from people in our medical humanities group may reveal some of the differences in response: the first person has some literature background and sees 'literature' on medical topics first and foremost as literature, as imaginative writing that can have a social effect in a broad sense. The second person, from an exclusively medical background, was more focused on the function of literature in a specifically medical context. Both points of view are valuable and we have found this mix of backgrounds productive; it has helped us not to translate every text into a set of learning outcomes.

These literary texts have kept us learning, presenting us with verbal puzzles and prompting us to debatable interpretations. Medical humanities has worked for us as a mode of continuing professional development: it has helped us to develop new skills:

New skills

Verbal interpretation
Listening
Interacting with those who hold different views
Talking about difficult issues
Sifting personal beliefs from professional codes of practice
and developing a view on a topic about which there is on-going debate in the media (like HRT, at the time of writing, 1996).

This continuing professional development effect is as yet unmeasured, even undefined, and its impact on people's professional practice is unknown. Periodic discussion of this very point, we have found, does allow people to take stock, but since **private** writing is our core activity on this kind of question, there has been no 'accounting' of the total effect. Semi-structured questionnaires in the Glasgow group and the Roadshow have provided the illustrations of a range of views presented earlier in these introductory chapters. I included them because I feel that they illustrated the variety of views that is the group's strength. And this is the dramatic effect of a literary text; it can produce as many interpretations as there are people in the room. For each individual there are the complementary outcomes of narration and reflection.

Narration, in this context, is taken to mean giving an account of a sequence of events which actually happened, drawing on recall and perhaps therefore factual. This account may closely or loosely relate to the subject of the literary text. It may also involve drawing on professional experience, and justifying a judgement based on that experience. Indicators of narration, in discussions, are usually along the following lines:

> That happened to me when ...
> That's what I would usually do ...
> I remember a case of ...
> What she probably means is ...
> What would probably happen is ...
> When I worked in Australia we used to ....

Reflection, by contrast, refers to commenting, evaluating, critiquing, consolidating, and is perhaps less tied to factual experience. Its indicators might take one of the following forms:

> I wonder if ...
> What might have happened if ...?
> I could have done ...
> What do you think of ...?
> Is that the same thing as ...?

Usually, in medical humanities, narration is readily forthcoming, in abundance, particularly if there is a desire to 'educate' the literary specialist and other non-medical people in the group about the medical subject or context. Reflection may take a bit of prompting, through reference to the text.

The balance of narration and reflection would be an interesting subject of study. Both can complement each other, bringing together actual, factual events and imaginative, speculative statements. Using writing prompts, for writing activities, can encourage both kinds of writing, if both kinds of prompt are used. This is a useful way to ensure that both narration and reflection do take place. Ideally, in other words, there should be both.

As people respond and interact, using both narration and reflection, it is interesting to note down what they say. This may in fact make it easier to assess what is taking place, i.e. to consider during or after the discussion what the balance of narration and reflection is. These notes can be also used as prompts for future discussions.

Complementary outcomes: personal and professional observations

---

In each section in this chapter I try to capture an aspect of medical humanities. I have tried to express its creative spark and its potential for pushing us to develop both our views and our ways of expressing them. I have tried to argue for the inclusion of medical humanities in undergraduate education and in postgraduate training without arguing too much against the status quo.

Clearly, for medical humanities to have any effect you have to have some goal like improving communication skills, developing a holistic approach, improving clinical skills or enjoying reading more literature. Equally clearly, most undergraduate and postgraduate curricula will include educational objectives like these. It's just that medical humanities is a new way of achieving them.

There are also personal outcomes, since the individual imagination will have been touched by a literary text: enjoyment, wonder at a writer's verbal skills, at the power of an apt image, the mystery of a complex line, the cleverness of deliberate ambiguity, and the trick of turning painful experience into beautiful writing.

The professional or educational outcomes can complement the personal outcomes. Neither is foregrounded in our medical humanities group, and both personal and professional responses are prompted by a creative text on the subject of one's profession. There is, therefore, potential for achieving both without removing any topics from the curriculum, without taking a formal course and without spending a lot of money. (We have agreed, in our group, an annual subscription of £20 to cover costs.)

3 Overview of texts

Literary texts ● *Non-literary texts* ● *Conclusion*

Literary texts

Over the past 5 years we have used poems, short stories and extracts from novels and plays. All of the texts we used were short, in order to allow for detailed discussion and so that it would be feasible for participants to make time to read them.

I included a variety of forms of writing: literature written in English from the USA – e.g. Walt Whitman, Adrienne Rich, May Sarton, Michael Crichton; from Scotland – e.g. Edwin Morgan, Janice Galloway, George Mackay Brown, Candia McWilliam; and from England – e.g. Elizabeth Jennings. We read literature from the 19th and 20th centuries, from 'high' and 'popular' culture and written by women and by men. We also included non-published writing.

We also found a wealth of material in anthologies of, for example, poems on medical topics. A selection of these texts is presented in Chapters 5–10, with full details of possible directions for discussion.

Selective overview

This chapter provides a selective overview in order to give an impression of the range of these writers' frames of reference and perhaps to prompt readers to produce their own examples.

Examples

This section gives examples of literary texts, while the next section gives examples of non-literary texts, although these two kinds of writing do overlap. Similarly, the line between fiction and biography is sometimes blurred.

May Sarton's *After the Stroke* is a journal in which she documents her illness and her feelings about it. As a first-hand account it provides both her version of a medical record and a personal record of her emotional responses to the stroke, including her almost paralysing fear of the changes that the stroke will bring:

Sunday, June 15
Will the time come when I can listen to Mozart again? What keeps me from playing records, like a finger across my mouth? The fear of a complete howling crack-up? Or that poetry would then seize me and shake me to pieces like a wild animal with prey? Who knows?
Sarton, M. (1988) *After the Stroke: A Journal*, Women's Press, London, p. 50

Robbie Kydd's *Auld Zimmery* is also told from the point of view of the person experiencing care. An 'auld' (old) man offers his view of the world, recalling the past but also reflecting on himself in the present, showing the weakness of his memory and the strength of his sense of humour. He, too, recognizes changes in himself that interfere with what he takes to be the meaning of the word 'living':

'Time passes. Listen. Time passes.' Curly-headed what's-his-name, died of drink, I can't remember. No matter how hard I listen I can't keep track of time passing. Sometimes it goes fast, sometimes slow. Sometimes it seems to stop altogether, but I don't die. I just exist, taking a minimal part in the routine of living, if 'living' is the word. When I write down a happening in this diary I can't place it on any kind of time-scale, so I've given up putting in dates. They're meaningless. When Fiona says 'last week' she might as well say 'last year'....
Just writing about that woman makes my heart pump to overload, so I stop and lie down under my duvet and fall asleep like a good boy. A more-or-less good boy. A bad boy, to be honest. But bad boys sleep as soundly as good boys, so I sleep well.   Kydd, R. (1987) *Auld Zimmery*, Mariscat, Glasgow, pp. 18-19

Douglas Dunn's collection of poems, *Elegies*, charts the diagnosis, decline and death of his wife from cancer. He mingles his own grief and her pain in his description of their last weeks together. Verbal snapshots detail their preparations for her death:

Each day was duty round the clock.
Our kissing conversations kept me going,
Those times together with the phone switched off,
Remembering our lives by candlelight.
Dunn, D. (1985) *Elegies*, Faber, London, p. 14

The different routes, or 'doors', to death are the subject of George Mackay Brown's poem 'The Door of Water'. Here death is viewed in abstract, symbolic terms. Each finds his/her own symbolic exit, and the whole creates a sense less of the violence of death and more of the pattern of our collective deaths:

Think of death, how it has many doors.
A child enters the Dove Door

And leaves a small wonderment behind.
For airmen there is the Door of Fire.
Most of us, with inadequate heart or lung or artery,
Disappear through the simple Door of the Skull.

Brown, G. M. (1976) *Winterfold*, Hogarth Press, London, p. 30

In much more physical terms, Robert Burns expresses first-hand the pain of toothache in his 'Address to the Toothache Written When the Author was Grievously Tormented by That Disorder'. He describes his experience in terms of a violent assault:

My curse upon thy venom'd stang,
That shoots my tortured gums alang;
And through my lugs gies mony a twang,
Wi' gnawing vengeance;
Tearing my nerves wi' bitter pang,
Like racking engines!

Burns, R. (1969) *Poems and Songs*, (ed. J. Kinsley), Oxford University Press, Oxford, p. 624

stang = sting; alang = along; lugs gies mony = ears gives many

The physical details of various illnesses are described in Dominique Lapierre's novel *City of Joy*, combining fact and fiction in 'faction'. What he conveys is his sense of shock at an overwhelming array of what were for him new health problems in India. In this case, then, we have the physician's view of illnesses, combining his professional observations of 'manifestations' and his personal reaction to the responsibility of having to deal with them:

Max Loeb was out of his depth, drowned, submerged. Nothing he had learned at school had prepared him for this confrontation with the physiological poverty of the Third World at its very worst. Manifestations such as eyes that were extremely yellow, chronic weight loss, painfully swollen ganglions in the throat corresponded with nothing he knew or recognized. Yet these were the symptoms of the most widespread disease in India, the one that caused by far the highest mortality: tuberculosis.

Lapierre, D. (1986) *City of Joy*, Arrow Books, London, p. 344

Janice Galloway's *The Trick is to Keep Breathing* documents the main character's breakdown. Innovative textual devices convey her point of view. For example, interjections interrupt the on-going narrative to convey her thoughts – 'HAH'. This novel shows us the character attempting simultaneously to construct a coherent narrative and to show her scorn for such coherence, hence the combination of black humour and panic:

I said, I'm no use with strangers.
He said, But this is different. Health Visitors are trained to cope with that. He said she would know what to do; she would find me out and make me talk.
Make me talk.
HAH

I'm putting on the kettle, still catching my breath when she comes in without knocking and frightens me. What if I had been saying things about her out loud? I tell her to sit in the living room so I can have time to think.
Tray

jug

sweeteners

plates

cups and saucers

another spoon

christ

the biscuits
the biscuits.

Galloway, J. (1992) *The Trick is to Keep Breathing*, Minerva, London, p. 20

Like Galloway, Candia McWilliam shows the effects, without explaining the cause or name, of an illness in her novel *A Little Stranger*, told from the point of view of the woman suffering from a disease that is not named until the end of the novel. It is a powerful study of the process of denial and of the workings of the illness itself. But since the illness is only hinted at throughout most of the novel there is a sense of mystery, which dramatizes the experience of living with the disease, or of living with someone who suffers from it. The reader is never allowed to be absolutely sure if there is a physical problem, a psychological problem or both. Even the question of which character suffers from it remains unanswered. Further uncertainty is created by the illusion that we are being taken into the character's confidence, a case of the patient's point of view representing vividly their experience but having to be taken with a pinch of salt, so to speak.

Note the bitter, yet playful, irony of 'served' in a narrative about eating disorders. Note also how the reader is apparently involved in the narrative, addressed as 'you', creating a sense that we have the facts, although in fact the first-hand account is still ambiguous. Note the use of 'Bries', the plural of Brie cheese, a noun we rarely, I think, use or see in the plural:

The only full description of a work of eating I have served you so far was when I described to you the blue and white bowls of nuts, laid out after supper. Enough to keep ... What is it nannies say? Enough to starve the feeding millions ...

My hogging began in joy. I was a pig in muck. Not two, not four, but ten of everything. I moved with the times; I was a decimal eater....

At its height, the midnight feasting was Dutch, wanting only an urn of tulips to freeze it to still life. I arranged cold fowl (which I ate, wrenching like a midwife with my hands) and sausages with flecks of white fat. On pewter dishes I dumped clouds of bread and flitches of striped speck. Transparent red smoked beef hung over plates, silky as poppy petals. I tumbled grapes from blue to yellow and the weak purple of primulas. I cushioned myself with Bries rich as white velvet. All this in trencherly quantities.

It was so beautiful; how could it do harm?
At the same time, Margaret was carrying out her inverted worship of the same
god.   McWilliam, C. (1989) *A Little Stranger*, Picador, London, pp. 127–128

The tension between stories, even personal journals, and experience is explored by Adrienne Rich in her poem 'Diving into the Wreck'. She explores the power of myths, using imagery of underwater diving to represent the risk and power of personal experience:

> I came to explore the wreck....
> I came to see the damage that was done ...
> the thing I came for:
> the wreck and not the story of the wreck
> the thing itself and not the myth
> the drowned face always staring
> toward the sun
> the evidence of damage
> worn by salt and sway into this threadbare beauty.
>
> Rich, A. (1984) *The Fact of a Doorframe, Poems Selected and New*, 1950–1984,
> Norton, London, pp. 163–164

The tension between myth and experience, and the effort required to separate the two, in this poem added another dimension to our discussion of hormone replacement therapy (HRT). In this poem myth is represented as sometimes having the power to drive out both knowledge and experience. An apparently tenuous link between these readings was made much stronger in the course of our discussion, particularly when some women in the group revealed their experiences of HRT: as a group we discovered in our discussion that a mixture of myth and scientific 'fact' surrounds HRT, so that some of Rich's lines about myth seemed to ring true for some women's experience of HRT:

> We are, I am, you are
> by cowardice or courage
> the one who finds our way
> back to this scene
> carrying a knife, a camera
> a book of myths
> in which
> our names do not appear.   p. 164

Summary

- These literary texts all have in common a medical subject, with a very wide range of meanings for the word 'medical'.
- This is just a selection of texts we used in our group; there are many more.

- The aim of this section is to illustrate the variety of readings, with potential talking points about each one.
- This selection may well prompt readers to add other texts to this list of medical humanities readings.

Non-literary texts

Readers might expect this selection of non-literary texts to include more facts and documentation; in fact, many of these readings are based on particular points of view or on stated standpoints in debates.

We do not use non-literary texts on their own in our discussions; we always include literary texts. We look at a non-literary text not as a factual or 'correct' account but as a presentation of a particular point of view.

This section again aims to illustrate the variety of texts that can be used in medical humanities, along with some of the talking points they provoked in our group.

In *Able Lives* women document their experience of traumatic spinal injury and the adjustments it requires. First-hand accounts reveal an impression of the medical profession, in the form of a disappointed expectation that they would help the women to make that adjustment:

While a few of us praised the excellent treatment received, more were critical of the care, rehabilitation and general support that was expected in these centres. One particular criticism, common among women of all ages, was that there was little or no help in coming to terms with the emotional upheaval caused by the trauma of sudden paralysis. Some of us highlighted this as the only fault in an otherwise satisfactory rehabilitation, but for others this problem affected the whole experience of hospitalization. The failure to address the emotional aspects of our injury was also associated with other criticisms which centred around the way in which women's concerns were ignored, the quality of care and a failure to help us plan our future.

Morris, J. (ed.) (1989) *Able Lives: Women's Experience of Paralysis*, Women's Press, London, p. 23

We found articles on health issues in the health section (often the women's page, for some reason) of national newspapers or in special features on specific topical subjects. For example, one national newspaper article gave tips on how to be a good visitor, but in doing so also raised questions about the conventions of care in hospitals – a topic ripe for debate:

In certain non-Western cultures, it is customary for patients in hospital to be largely tended and cared for by relatives who literally camp beside the bed. Whether this is in response to a shortage of nurses or a cultural norm, the effect is the same – the patient is surrounded by familiar people at a profoundly stressful time. Significantly, the family have a defined role in the care of their loved one and a medium through which to express their concern.

The Herald, **5.2.91**, p. 10

Susan Sontag's mixture of linguistic and sociological commentary unravels the mystique surrounding our most popular and deadly illnesses: TB, cancer and, more recently, AIDS. She exposes what she calls the 'punitive or sentimental fantasies' which, she argues, we have created around these diseases:

Although the way in which disease mystifies is set against a backdrop of new expectations, the disease itself (once TB, cancer today) arouses thoroughly old-fashioned kinds of dread. Any disease that is treated as a mystery and acutely enough feared will be felt to be morally, if not literally, contagious. Thus, a surprisingly large number of people with cancer find themselves being shunned by relatives and friends and are the objects of practices of decontamination by members of their household, as if cancer, like TB, were an infectious disease.

Sontag, S. (1977) *Illness as Metaphor*, Penguin, Harmondsworth, pp. 9–10

Oliver Sachs, in *Awakenings*, mingles medical study and personal commentary, including a critique of the medical establishment which rejected his results, both on the grounds of his method and his style of presentation. His aim, in writing about his cases, was not to represent an external point of view, but to represent the patients' experience of the illness:

The general style of this book – with its alternation of narrative and reflection, its proliferation of images and metaphors, its remarks, repetitions, asides, and footnotes – is one which I have been impelled towards by the very nature of the subject-matter. My aim is not to make a system, or to see patients as systems, but to picture a world, a variety of worlds – the landscapes of being in which these patients reside. And the picturing of worlds requires not a static and systematic formulation, but an active exploration of images and views, a continual jumping-about and imaginative movement.

Sachs, O. (1990) *Awakenings*, Picador, London, p. xviii

Writing by patients offers direct insights into their points of view: cardiac rehabilitation participants were invited to write about their experience, to write about themselves before and after their MI. Many saw this as an opportunity to thank their carers; others chose to write about the radical changes they saw in themselves since their MI:

Before January 16th 1987, Saturdays were shopping days, feet up in the evenings, and admitting to smoking 20 a day. Since my heart attack, Saturdays have, weather permitting – and sometimes despite it – become the high spot of the week, rambling over the Kilpatrick Hills with my wife, home to hot baths and cool salads, and feet up in the evenings.   Unpublished

Strenuous debate is repeatedly provoked by the newsletter *What Doctors Don't Tell You*, which has as its stated aim, perhaps clearly enough from the title, to tell us 'what every doctor knows ... about drugs that could harm you, surgery you don't need, diagnostic tests that are unreliable and everyday treatments that are untested ... but didn't get around to telling you. Plus, a few things he [sic] doesn't know about' (publicity leaflet for *WDDTY*).

Specific topics dealt with in separate issues of this newsletter, some running over several issues are: allergies, amalgam fillings, antibiotics, *Candida albicans*, child health care, HRT, immunization, ME, tranquillizers, etc. In addition, non-mainstream books on medical topics, particularly on topics that are the subject of widespread debate, are frequently reviewed in this newsletter, making it a source, for us, of further readings.

Chapman & Hall's series on non-clinical skills has provided up-to-date examples of good practice which in themselves can be the raw material for debate and discussion. For example, in a concluding chapter to *Communicating with Patients*, Phillip Ley presents findings of a patient survey on satisfaction with communications. His implicit point about being tutored rather than 'untutored' on this topic raised a number of questions:

Satisfaction with communications

The main findings about satisfaction with communications are as follows.

(a) Satisfaction with the communications aspect of the consultation correlates highly with satisfaction with other aspects of the clinician–patient interaction.

(b) Substantial numbers of patients feel dissatisfied with the communications aspect of their clinical encounters. This contrasts with unusually high levels of satisfaction with other aspects of the clinician–patient interaction.

(c) This dissatisfaction does not seem to be reduced by clinicians trying (in untutored ways) to see that patients are fully informed.

(d) The increase in educational and research concern with the problem, which has taken place over the last two decades, does not seem to have led to a reduction in levels of patients' dissatisfaction.

Ley, P. (1988) *Communicating with Patients*, Chapman & Hall, London, pp. 172–173

'Storied therapy' also seemed so relevant to our medical humanities work that we included it in our discussion. This approach encourages creative writing, in structured ways, and we were able to try some of this in our group, in the form of private writing, and then to discuss its impact on us and its potential for education and training. We took White and Epstein's section on the practice of storied therapy as our starting point for both our writing and our discussion:

A therapy situated within the context of the narrative mode of thought would take a form that:

1. privileges the person's lived experience;
2. encourages a perception of a changing world through the plotting or linking of lived experience through the temporal dimension;
3. invokes the subjunctive mood in the triggering of presuppositions, the establishment of implicit meaning, and in the generation of multiple perspective;
4. encourages polysemy [use of variety of language] and the use of ordinary, poetic and picturesque language in the description of experience and in the endeavour to construct new stories.

White, M. and Epstein, D. (1990) *Narrative Means to Therapeutic Ends*, Norton, New York, p. 83

These are four of eight points that outline the mode of storied therapy which we adapted in a private writing task in our group.

Finally, we also discussed different ways of writing about science. There are now many varieties of scientific works written for a wide audience and specialist texts and journals that aspire to Plain English. And there are those who have missed or rejected revolutions in scientific writing and would think it radical and disruptive to begin a sentence with 'and'. For example, 'Can scientific discovery be premeditated?' is a provocative essay, in plain English, in which Medawar explores underlying assumptions about 'the scientific method':

Most of the day-to-day business of science consists in making observations or experiments designed to find out whether this imagined world of our hypotheses corresponds to the real one. An act of imagination, a speculative adventure, thus underlies every improvement of natural knowledge.

Medawar, P. (1984) *The Limits of Science*, Oxford University Press, Oxford, p. 51

Medawar uses three examples of scientific discoveries, X-rays, HLA polymorphism and the nature of myasthenia gravis (MG), 'that could not have been the specific outcome of a conscious and declared attempt to make them' (p. 45), thus questioning certain assumptions some scientists hold dear. (This essay has provoked interesting discussions among undergraduate physics students.)

Similarly, the abstractions of science are made more accessible by Gribbin, whose *In Search of Schrödinger's Cat* tackles quantum theory in plain English, in a combination of simple language (p. 1), abstract language (p. 2, p. 3) and technical language (p. 215):

Without quantum mechanics, chemistry would still be in the Dark Ages and there would be no science of molecular biology – no understanding of DNA, no genetic engineering – at all.... For what quantum mechanics says is that nothing is real and that we cannot say anything about what things are doing when we are not looking at them.... Nothing is real unless it is observed.... The direct, experimental proof of the paradoxical reality of the quantum world comes from modern versions of the EPR experiment. The modern experiments don't involve measurements of the position and momentum of particles, but of spin and polarization.

> Gribbin, J. (1984) *In Search of Schrödinger's Cat*, Corgi, London, pp. 1–3, 215

Like Medawar, Gleick questions the traditional notion of 'the' scientific method in an account of the development of chaos theory as developing from one of the mathematical methods, also using simple language:

A researcher picks up a problem and begins by making a decision about which way to continue. It happened that often that decision involved a choice between a path that was mathematically feasible and a path that was interesting from the point of view of understanding nature. For a mathematician, the choice was clear: he [sic] would abandon any obvious connection with nature for a while.

> Gleick, J. (1987) *Chaos, Making a New Science*, Abacus, London, p. 89

Gleick also humanizes the theoretical and complex subject by using short narratives about the people who first developed it:

One wintry afternoon in 1975, aware of the parallel currents emerging in physics, preparing his first major work for publication in book form, Mandelbrot decided he needed a name for his shapes, his dimensions, and his geometry. His son was home from school, and Mandelbrot found himself thumbing through the boy's Latin dictionary. He came across the adjective *fractus*, from the verb *frangere*, to break. The resonance of the main English cognates – *fracture* and *fraction* – seemed appropriate. Mandelbrot created the word ... *fractal*.

> p. 98

Conclusion

This overview is intended to illustrate, above all, the range of literary and non-literary texts which we have used in our medical humanities group. We have consciously tried to include both 'great' literature – the literature of the English departments' curricula – and popular and contemporary writers. We have tried deliberately to maintain variety in the readings.

In my role as group facilitator I have also been conscious of the need to break down the mystique of published writing by asking participants to do some writing themselves, in the form of private writing for discussion, at least once during each session. In this way they find out, in discussion with other members of the group, not only that their own writing can be just as interesting but also, even more surprising, that it can be enjoyable and stimulating to do.

The distinction between 'literary' and 'non-literary' texts is perhaps open to question: new forms of scientific writing, appealing to a wider audience, have adopted new styles. The new science and new maths have also adapted traditional methods and assumptions. For some readers this blurs the distinction between the humanities and the sciences. Indeed, the interaction of the two can reveal surprising similarities. All the more reason for both forms of text, both kinds of interpretation, to be included in our education and our continuing development.

The breadth of the selection in this chapter, finally, is designed to encourage readers to look for medical humanities in a variety of places and in a variety of forms.

4 Overview of methods

The theme approach ● *Issues for debates:* ● *Daily dilemmas or 'minor to major'* ● *Conclusion to Part One: to what end?*

This is what we do

This chapter gives an overview of methods that have emerged in our medical humanities group; this is therefore by no means a comprehensive list of methods. Since the primary aim of this book is to enable readers to participate in their own groups, this chapter does not present theoretical models of medical humanities but patterns of discussion that emerged in practice in our group and have been tried with other groups. With these possibilities for discussion in mind the facilitator can allow the discussion to drift and look out for emerging themes. Alternatively, the discussion can be steered towards themes, depending on the style of the group.

The key to our approach is that it has been open and varied. The lack of any fixed agenda, the lack of a unifying theme, the lack of even continuity of venue has helped us to preserve spontaneity and variety in the discussions. These features make it very different from other educational experiences. Nor does continuing professional development usually offer this kind of extended open discussion among mixed groups.

Unpredictability is a feature of our discussions: it is not possible to predict how a discussion will go or even how people you know well will respond to certain texts. To some extent Part Two of this book does begin to set an agenda for several meetings, but options for routes for discussion and notes on the varieties of comment people are likely to make are also provided. Those chapters can be used as a starting point, rather than an agenda, by those who feel confident enough to let the discussion roam freely.

This chapter has three sections:

● the first defines the 'theme' approach, which involves bringing together several texts on one topic;

- the second defines an issues-based method, which involves identifying topical, or recurring, 'issues for debates';
- the third defines a 'daily dilemmas' approach, which involves attending to issues raised by participants, relating to their own experience or practice.

The theme approach

What is the 'theme approach'?

Theme: the subject of discourse, discussion, conversation, meditation or composition; a topic.   *Shorter Oxford English Dictionary*

The theme approach in medical humanities simply means taking three or four texts, medical or scientific and non-medical or non-scientific, which are loosely or closely connected by subject matter. This connection can be either explicit or implicit; it can be either a starting point for discussion, adding focus, or one of its possible outcomes. Ultimately, if members of the group are not interested in the theme there is always the option of focusing on whatever has emerged as a focus in the course of discussion.

Using the theme approach, texts can be selected for their common subject matter, thus explicitly exploring a theme. Alternatively, unforeseen connections between texts can emerge in discussion, thus revealing a theme. In our group we have used both approaches, acknowledging that some issues recur in many of our discussions whichever approach we adopt.

We have found that some topics emerge and recur over several discussions. These, then, have developed as themes particular to our group: power, institutionalization, control, the patient's point of view, time, and the medical model of care. Whatever the topic, the issue of power seems to appear in every discussion. We have returned to a number of key questions about power:

Power: a recurring theme

Who makes the decisions?
Who can make changes?
What are the patient's rights?
Why do patients not ask for more?

Here is one example of the theme approach in practice. These four texts were chosen because they deal with the topic – ageing – in very different ways. This collection of literary and non-literary texts reveals common issues such as change, illness and loss. Placing these texts together reveals striking contrasts between scientific and literary approaches to the subject.

Example of a theme: ageing

1.

Most people at 65 can look forward to a dozen years of good health, a few much longer. Most people require substantial care in the last six months to a year of their lives. Care givers need the virtue of **humility** as an antidote to their arrogance of power. They are receivers, as well as givers, in the professional relationship. It goes without saying that care receivers also need the same virtue. The progressive loss of friends, job, bodily prowess and energy, the passing look on the faces of the young that tells us we are old – these experiences assault one's dignity: they humiliate. All the care in the world will not overcome the sting of humiliation; only humility can.

May, W. F. (1985) The virtues and vices of the elderly. *Socio-Economic Planning Sciences (Special Issue)*, **19**(4), 258

2.

The ageing process produces quite obvious external bodily changes, such as hair loss and wrinkling of the skin, and there are observable functional changes such as failing eyesight, hearing and agility, all of which affect the quality of life. An acquaintance trying to describe being old to my young son, asked him to imagine having his glasses smeared with Vaseline, cotton wool stuck in his ears and walking with stones in his shoes!

Fallowfield, L. (1990) The Quality of Life: The Missing Measurement in Health Care, Souvenir Press, London, p. 168

3.

When the cardioversion finally took place I was anaesthetized for a few seconds and it was over. Dr Petrovich said, 'It's fine. It's done the trick!' Euphoria! I was a prisoner set free. And for an hour I lay there in bliss waiting for a sandwich and a glass of milk – it was near two.

But then when a nurse brought me the pill, Amiodoroni [sic], the one that makes me ill, I realized I was being asked to go back to hell. It was a traumatic reversal and a storm of tears popped out of me. Late that night, around nine-thirty, after I had gone to sleep, now in a private room with the same lovely view I had had before of a line of trees against the sky, Dr Petrovich came in. Yes, I have to take the pill or have another stroke. The hardest thing psychologically to take is that he does not believe this drug makes me sick.

Sarton, M. (1988) After the Stroke: A Journal, Women's Press, London, p. 51

4.

'Still writing rubbish?' asks Fiona, when she finds me dozing upright in my bed, my A4 pad and my trusty 0.7 Pentel still in my hand, implying that writing is a poor way of coming alive, but better than nothing. I could try harder.
'Aye,' I reply, wide awake at her challenge.
'Kin I read it?'
'Well. Yes. I suppose so,' I temporize, thinking she may be growing up, actually asking my permission, but there's dynamite in some of the complaints I've made about this place and its denizens. Could she handle all that and not clype? I look into her face uncertainly and its expression is unfamiliar. Something must have happened to her. She's a shade less hard and sulky, almost vulnerable. Her ears look naked with her hair shaved away at the sides like that, but they are shapely ears; worth showing off, but vulnerable. I hand her the pad, after flipping back the pages to the place where I want her to start. She reads my scrawl rather slowly, moving her lips. She looks up.

Kydd, R. (1987) *Auld Zimmery*, Mariscat, Glasgow, p. 15

aye = yes, Kin I = can I, clype = tell tales

What is the approach to ageing in each of these texts? Each text has a different audience and purpose. The point of view is different in each one. There are different assumptions about the experience of ageing behind each treatment of the subject. Our reactions to each text are shaped by how it is written. For example, some readers will find the role of 'humility' in the first reading a little overstated, while others will find it useful for their practice and in their caring for ageing relatives. One wonders how the characters, carer and old man, in the fourth reading would respond to this appeal for their humility: 'Still writing rubbish? ... there's dynamite in some of the complaints I've made about this place'.

What does the placing together of these texts achieve? What is the effect of the comparison? Assumptions about the subject are more starkly revealed in the placing together of these four writings. We can see differences between the generalized accounts and the first-hand accounts. We can then consider the implications of these differences. The texts can then be used as points of reference in a discussion of different approaches to ageing:

1. an abstract, socio-philosophical approach;
2. a factual, generalized approach;
3. a first-hand account of the side-effects of ageing;
4. a first-hand account of rebellion against it.

These texts could also be defined in terms of their target audiences, the first two most easily, the other two having a broader appeal but with differences in the treatment of age, gender and class affecting the readership:

1. sociologists of health, academics;
2. health professionals, students;
3. general public, biographical interest;
4. general public.

In comparing these texts the group could consider the implications of obvious and subtle differences between them. There are many points of comparison, which would reveal the personal, professional and political agendas that have, in a sense, shaped each text:

- Point of view shapes content.
- Emotional responses to ageing can be included or excluded.
- Relationships can be explored.
- Mechanisms of power in institutions can be explored.
- Certainty and uncertainty can be revealed, in terms of both the view stated and the way in which it is stated.

For example, we could compare specific word choices in two texts and consider how word choice shapes our interpretation. A comparison between text 1 – which takes what I have called an abstract, socio-philosophical approach to the subject of ageing – and text 4 – which I have called a first-hand account of rebellion against ageing – reveals different levels of certainty:

Table 4.1 Comparison of texts 1 and 4

Text 1: Certain	Text 4: Uncertain
'Most people ...Most people require... It goes without saying that ...'	'I look into her face... uncertainly and its expression is unfamiliar'.

Moreover, these comparisons can raise issues about the relative status of different texts; particularly the question: What does the literary text do – in these examples – that the non-literary text does not?

Why use the theme approach? It is possible that focusing on one topic, in several readings, has a particular effect on discussion:

- focusing discussion on a particular topic;
- enabling participants to engage with a literary text if they know about the topic;
- prompting deeper discussion of one topic;
- allowing different sides in the debate to be represented in the readings;
- holding the discussion together;
- providing continuity to participants' initial and final writings during discussion.

Themes: some examples

A list of examples of themes we have used in our discussions is given below. These were not generated by our group on demand or in advance; these did not by any means shape our discussions. Instead, these were the themes that emerged over months as issues that seemed to concern us most, since they kept recurring in our discussions. Other groups may find that they have other concerns, so that this list may be no more than a useful starting point:

Death and dying
Ageing
Cancer
Power
Gender
Disability
Sexuality
Institutionalization.

Issues for debates

The 'big issues'

The group can list a number of topics that interest them. Individuals can identify a topic which interests them and the facilitator can then select texts which deal with that topic. For example, topics which participants have identified in our group are:

The 'big issues'

Abortion
Bullying
Euthanasia
Health policy
Ways of dying
Feminist analysis
Discrimination
Hormone replacement therapy
Complementary Medicine
Genetic engineering
and

Whatever medical subject is topical, in the media.

Daily dilemmas or 'minor to major'

Issues that come up in discussion are often related to professional practice. In discussion we have found that the ideals of practice can be compromised by local circumstances. This can be highly frustrating for the individual. The focus of the discussion can quickly shift from the big issues of the day – like genetic engineering – to the apparently relatively small issues of everyday – like the time carers can give to each patient.

Since these daily dilemmas, as we have called them, occur repeatedly and have no apparent resolution they can be even more important to the individual carer and patient. The daily dilemmas that have come up in our discussions are:

Daily dilemmas

Whistle blowing
Audit
Doing research
Asserting yourself and/or your profession
Communicating
The health-care team dynamic
Management styles
Time constraints.

These are topics which we find crop up again and again as we discuss the texts. Unlike the 'big issues', reference to these daily dilemmas can be triggered by any text; they seem to be universal, relevant to any text, any medical experience. If a group or individual continues to refer repeatedly to one or more of these, it might seem to get a bit 'old'. However, we have found that it is possible to work through some of these issues, at least to the extent of having our say. Perhaps these issues could best be seen as a thread, a kind of undercurrent running through all of our discussions. Perhaps this is because each of these daily dilemmas exposes our values-in-action?

Conclusion to Part One: to what end?

What is the effect of medical humanities?: how do you know it works?
Does it improve clinical practice?: where is the evidence?
Does it produce personal/professional development?: measured as ...?

These are questions which remain unanswered in the literature. Various claims have been made for medical humanities:

Five broad goals are met by including the study of literature in medical education: 1) Literary accounts of illness can teach physicians concrete and powerful lessons about the lives of sick people; 2) great works of fiction about medicine enable physicians to recognize the power and implications of what they do; 3) through the study of narrative, the physician can better understand patients' stories of sickness and his or her own personal stake in medical practice; 4) literary study contributes to physicians' expertise in narrative ethics; and 5) literary theory offers new perspectives on the work and the genres of medicine.

Charon, R. et al. (1995) Literature and medicine: contributions to clinical practice. Annals of Internal Medicine, 122, 599

It has been claimed that medical humanities offers possibilities for strengthening students' and practitioners' ability to 'recognize the human dimensions of all of the experiences that occur within their gaze' (Charon et al., 1995, p. 604). Moreover, these authors, based in what was one of the first Departments of Medical Humanities in the United States at Pennsylvania State University (which made the first appointment in Medical Humanities in a US medical faculty), having worked with medical humanities for over 20 years, have clarified conceptual frameworks and competencies which they have observed developing through the use of medical humanities in this context.

As yet, however, as they also document in this recent paper (1995) no one has been able to measure its effect. In fact, innovations in teaching and learning, in either undergraduate or postgraduate education, are notoriously difficult to measure. Perhaps 'measuring' is not possible using the quantitative methods implied by the word 'measure'. This difficulty is acknowledged in a number of recent papers and calculating the effect of medical humanities has been highlighted as a priority for future research:

The value of this course is neither easily measured nor easily stated.

Radwany, S. M. and Adelson, B. H. (1987) The use of literary classics in teaching medical ethics to physicians. Journal of the American Medical Association, 257 (12), 1631

Although research into the design, implementation and evaluation of PSL [problem-solving learning] in physiotherapy is indicated, no literature has been found which has investigated whether graduates of this new approach, as it exists in Britain, are more able than clinicians trained in the traditional way, in solving patients' problems, coping with the demands of modern professional practice or continuing their education.

Morris, J. (1993) An overview of and comparison among three current approaches to medical and physiotherapy undergraduate education. Physiotherapy, 79(2), 93

How do we know that teaching literature to physicians and medical students works? Outcome studies of literature and medicine courses have examined students' course evaluations, post-course interviews and questionnaires, and faculty members' assessments and have shown that such courses improve

students' understanding of patients' experiences, enrich students' capacities for dealing with ethical problems or deepen students' self-knowledge in clinically relevant ways....
Nevertheless, longitudinal outcome research is needed.

Charon, R. et al. (1995) Literature and medicine: contributions to clinical practice. Annals of Internal Medicine, **122**, 603–604

Perhaps the problem in evaluating medical humanities is that the effect of this kind of group work would be difficult to 'measure'. Perhaps qualitative research methods could be applied here, along the lines of the questions and quotations in Chapter 1, where information is gathered directly from participants over time in the kind of longitudinal study suggested by Charon et al. (1995). In this way outcomes could be defined. A theory of medical humanities could emerge. An assessment of its effects could be made.

As participants, in looking for effects, we should probably be clear about our expectations. Perhaps this could be a talking point in itself. Medical humanities does not make carers more caring. There is no essential meaning in the text or goal in the discussion that can only be uncovered by good detective work. Nor do we arrive at the idea that there is some essential experience or some essential 'humanity' to which all of us aspire. Over and above the fact that medical humanities is simply enjoyable, it can also prompt us to reflect on our practice and to interrogate some of our assumptions. A direct effect on our practice is therefore one of the possible outcomes, though it is questionable whether this is what motivates people to attend our group.

The format of this group has been open, *ad hoc*, aiming for variety in readings and across sessions, with input from participants, with no fixed agenda or format. Moreover, the group develops and changes over time: participants come and go. People's philosophies emerge over time, at their individual pace. Some find a particular attraction in turning up knowing that they will not agree with everything that is said in the discussion. This is a special kind of challenge. For some it is not found anywhere else. How do we measure the effect of that? This would certainly be an interesting area for further research.

As researchers we probably do need to come up with some answers to the questions about the effect of medical humanities, on a group, over time:

Is it really measurable?
Why should we measure it? How can we measure it?
Why should we assess this? How can we assess it?

This is the end of Part One of this book, in which the four introductory chapters were designed to answer some basic questions that medical humanities raises for those who have never come across it before. Part Two gives examples of medical humanities in practice, the aim here being to provide materials and methods that groups can use and adapt in their own discussion.

I would like to end Part One on a reassuring note: even those who have taken the plunge and done some medical humanities with very little experience of it themselves have found that students responded with enthusiasm and excitement. Likewise, when I have run one-off workshops with groups I have never met before they have also reacted positively. The debilitating mystique of 'literature' is diminished by the familiar medical subject. Most people are simply glad to be able to read literature again (with a semi-professional 'excuse').

Part Two : OUTLINES AND TEXTS FOR DISCUSSIONS

Part One of this book covered introductory material; its purpose was to define and illustrate medical humanities in general terms. Part Two is more specific, providing outlines and texts for specific medical humanities discussions.

These are examples that have been used with groups, and examples of their responses and reactions are also included.

The aim here is to provide sufficient material in sufficient detail for readers to run or participate in their own groups.

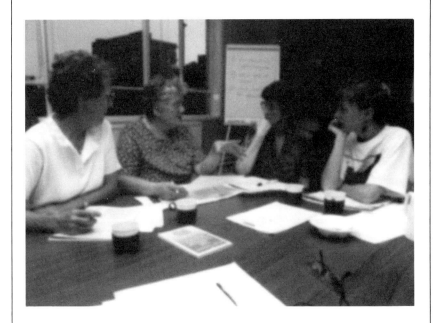

5 Getting started: 'After an Operation'

This chapter includes specific texts we have used and details of how we
used them in discussions. Topics discussed and responses produced by
participants in our medical humanities group are also provided to give
readers an indication of what to expect. The aim is to provide materials
that other groups, tutors or facilitators can use to generate their own
discussions.

While the specific directions of our discussions are given here, there
are also ideas for other directions.

The first meeting

When we first started a medical humanities group we were simply
enthusiastic to read some new, non-scientific, literature. We were also
struck by what we saw as an original approach. We were not sure what
it was an original approach to, but we knew we wanted to explore its
potential. It looked like an opportunity to explore alternative models
of care. We began to realize that this could mean exploring medical
subjects in all their complexities, including the human side of care.
Medical humanities could, we speculated, complement the medical
model of care.

What appealed to us most was the idea of bringing back some of the
art of medicine, something that was not proving possible in daily prac-

tice and was given little time, as we saw it, in education. Above all, we thought that medical humanities would be enjoyable. This is pretty much how we represented it to those who turned up to the first meeting, in terms of our own initial reactions:

Our starting point

This is something different.
It has potential.
We can read literature again.
What's it for? ... Does it need to have a purpose?
It's something I do for me – I enjoy this.

Advertising

The full text of our first poster was included in Chapter 2 (Fig. 2.1). We targeted selected hospital and university departments, hoping to attract a wide range of people: nurses, physiotherapists, doctors and others, including non-medical people. We specifically invited colleagues and friends whom we knew would be likely to take an interest in a new approach.

Since it was a completely new term, we felt we should offer a brief definition, both to explain and to arouse interest, combined with a brief example to illustrate the point:

What can the 'humanities' – literature, philosophy, etc. – tell us about medical care? Novels, short stories and poems can provide provocative insights and starting points for discussions of different views. For example, May Sarton's *After the Stroke* gives the patient's point of view of illness and treatments. Solzhenitsyn's *Cancer Ward* is another example of a work of literature which focuses on the medical world.

In this discussion group we will read extracts from works of literature and consider different experiences of health care, different medical conditions and their treatments and different views of the medical world.   Unpublished poster

Definitions

Since this was the first meeting, we also included in the readings two definitions of medical humanities. These quotations were chosen because they raise different kinds of question and give different insights:

Definitions

What is 'medical humanities'?

Medicine and art have a common goal: to complete what nature cannot bring to a finish ... to reach the ideal ... to heal creation. This is done by paying **attention**. The physician attends the patient; the artist attends nature.... If we are attentive in looking, in listening, and in waiting, then sooner or later something in the depths of ourselves will respond. Art, like medicine, is not an arrival; it's a search. This is why, perhaps, we call medicine itself an art.

> Breo, D. L. (1990) M. Therese Southgate, MD – the woman behind 'The Cover'.
> *Journal of the American Medical Association*, **263**(15), 2112

What is it for?

In *The Elephant Man*, dramatist Bernard Pomeranz draws a poignant picture of dignity in the face of overwhelming illness. Treves, the surgeon, and Merrick, the abused sideshow freak with neurofibromatosis, provide a powerful allegory for the relationship of physician to patient.
Course participants focused on the inherent irony of physicians' benefiting from their patients' suffering, as well as the potential for conflict of interest should that benefit become too great. Also explored was the inadvertent dehumanization of the most unfortunate patients, along with the conscious and unconscious denial of their sexuality. The physicians present examined their responses to certain 'types' of patients: The adversarial patient, the noble suffering patient, and the patient with an unavoidably poor outcome.

> Radwany, S. M. and Adelson, B. H. (1987) The use of literary classics in teaching
> medical ethics to physicians. *Journal of the American Medical Association*, **257**
> (12), 1630

The first quotation (Breo, 1990) makes great, perhaps abstract, claims, yet also reduces the acts of artist and physician to very human basics: 'paying attention ... looking ... listening ... waiting'. The comparison between the 'work of nature' and the 'work of medicine' and 'art', moreover, would be sure to challenge some people's views, and we were consciously trying to convey this stimulus to others from the start.

The second quotation (Radwany and Adelson, 1987) was chosen because it mentions a specific text, *The Elephant Man*, which some people would have heard of (or seen in the film version). In addition, it puts medical humanities in the context of a course, and this would make the idea more accessible, perhaps less threatening to some. Finally, Radwany has included an example of medical people discussing a literary subject and reflecting on their professional practice, thus providing the best kind of illustration of what we hoped we could do ourselves.

We also included a sample of possible topics for discussions, leaving it open-ended in order to invite participants to consider, and perhaps contribute, their own topics:

Possible topics for discussion

The body/the mind
Birth
Disability/handicap
Youth and age
Knowledge and uncertainty
Medical education
The pre-clinical curriculum
Hospitals
Whole-patient care
Doctors
Nurses
Physiotherapists
The patient's point of view

Others?

At the first meeting we invited participants to suggest specific texts we could read and discuss at future meetings – literary texts that dealt with a medical subject: poems, short stories, novels, articles, videos, films.

How to 'prep' the texts

What to look for in choosing a text? – a medical subject, in any sense of the word; a short text or extract, which can be read quickly; something which will provoke discussion, although it is important not to have any preconceptions about what people will actually say in the discussion. This will be fascinating; there will be surprises. If most or all participants contribute there will be a diversity of views.

Getting to know the text well in advance of the meeting is useful but there also needs to be freedom and flexibility in the discussion. A plan for the discussion is therefore not essential. It is far more important that the structure is clear (see below), that the questions are initially open, then focused (see below) and that the facilitator has the skills in group work to enable everyone to contribute. However, these chapters are intended to support newcomers to medical humanities: notes on each of the three texts for this session are therefore included here.

Notes on the extracts: talking points

Because this is the first meeting the agenda should be quite open and allow plenty of time for questions and discussion. However, it is a good idea to try to steer the discussion through phases of **initial reaction, discussion** and **further reflection**.

This structure can, of course, itself be open to question and discussion at the end of the session. Here are the extracts we read (or part of them, in the case of Sarton and Kydd), along with potential talking points on each text. Readers may not agree with all of the interpretations; these points should be seen as starting points, rather than endpoints, for discussion.

Texts

The texts we used in our first discussion were 'After an Operation', a poem by Elizabeth Jennings, and an extract from *After the Stroke: A Journal* by May Sarton. By way of introduction, these two are discussed here. I have also added an extract from the story *Auld Zimmery* by Robbie Kydd, to illustrate the development of a theme.

The first text, the poem 'After an Operation', was selected for the first meeting because it is immediately accessible. It is easy to read because its form and language are relatively simple and the emotions are clearly represented in emotional language: 'afraid ... frightened ... fear'. The poem also has a clear medical context, straight from the title: recuperation from an operation:

After an Operation

> What to say first? I learnt I was afraid
> Not frightened in the way that I had been
> When wide awake and well. I simply mean
> Fear became absolute and I became
> Subject to it; it beckoned, I obeyed.
>
> Fear which before had always been particular,
> Attached to this or that scene, word, event,
> Here became general. Past, future meant
> Nothing. Only the present moment bore
> This huge, vague fear, this wish for nothing more.
>
> Yet life still stirred and nerves themselves became
> Like shoots which hurt while growing, sensitive
> To find not death but further ways to live.
> And now I'm convalescent, fear can claim
> No general power. Yet I am not the same.
>
> Elizabeth Jennings

Notes: 'After an Operation'

The use of the first person – 'I' – shows first-hand experience, which proves useful in discussion. At first, it draws out personal responses in the group. Later, it makes us reflect on this personal response. Looking very closely at what the individual represented in the poem actually says helped us to see some of the differences between our interpretations and the first-hand experience.

The value of this poem as a starting point for medical humanities discussions was made even clearer when we used it in several sessions on our Medical Humanities Roadshow: several groups, including both those who knew each other and those who had never met, engaged in discussion of this text. We found it was effective in prompting discussion with a variety of groups, both among health professionals and among mixed groups. (This work is described in more detail in Murray and Thow, 1995.)

The poem begins with a question, 'What to say first?' Does this suggest uncertainty, or the first step in the process of putting things in order? The person in the poem has 'learnt' from an experience and seems, at this stage, to be taking stock of this learning. The experience of the operation seems to have created a new kind of fear; the experience of being ill has created a new kind of experience. As the person attempts to grapple with this new experience, the word 'simply' reveals the terms in which they choose to make sense of it: all the vocabulary in this verse is very simple. The last two lines in this verse, lines 4 and 5, convey the intensity of the fear this new experience has brought with it: 'Fear became absolute and I became/ Subject to it', and this is emphasized by restatement of the point, 'it beckoned, I obeyed' (line 5). The power of fear has taken up the whole of this first verse, one-third of the poem. However, 'I' has been persistently used throughout – to what effect? It appears six times in five lines. This conveys the individual's voice, as they wrestle with something 'absolute', but maintains the sense of a personal voice.

The second verse begins with the word 'Fear' and 'I' has disappeared. The next five lines, 6 to 10, describe its effects. Fear takes over at this stage and this represents the experience that is being described, where fear has swamped all other thoughts and perception. At the end of this verse, line 10, the fear is described as 'huge' and 'vague'. Over ten lines of the poem, therefore, fear has been described as 'absolute', 'general' and 'vague'. What do these words suggest? They convey the overall impact of the emotion, without using emotional words. The emotion of fear has taken over to the extent that it has not been pinned down in specific emotional terms. Perhaps this is the meaning of 'this wish for nothing more'? Is this where this kind of fear leaves a person, this person? The context of the 'operation', the hospital, has not been mentioned. Why is this? Why are there no references to carers or supporters? The focus is very much internal. Only the title tells us that the context is, or has been, a hospital. How has this fear become 'huge'?

At the start of the third verse the word 'Yet' signals a turn for the better. The imagery brings in the idea of a natural cycle – rebirth, new growth and recovery. The first three lines, 11–13, make this explicit; fear has been replaced by growth and now the threat of death can be replaced by the promise of life. There is a complete change of view here. The last two lines, 14 and 15, bring us back to the present tense with 'now' and the word 'convalescent', the first medical term in the poem, seems to put a clear label on this new phase. Significantly, the word 'I' reappears with this new phase and the power, and presence, of 'fear' is diminished. The final sentence in line 15 begins, like this third verse, with 'Yet' and therefore appears to turn away from the positive view of recovery: 'Yet I am not the same'. While this verse is predominantly positive, this final line clearly registers a sense of loss. This last sentence, very short, with simple, monosyllabic words, holds the poem finely balanced – 'Has this person fully recovered?'

Reactions to this poem were varied. Because the poem was used on the Medical Humanities Roadshow, including the Glasgow group, and at national and international conferences, I have had a wide range of answers to my question, 'Has this person fully recovered?' Details of these reactions, including direct quotations, are given later in this chapter. In my own re-readings of the poem, I have found that my answer to the question changes each time I read it.

The second text, May Sarton's *After the Stroke,* was chosen for a number of reasons: again, it presents the patient's point of view in a first-person account of the experience of illness; secondly, it was written by an American, and therefore came from a different context; thirdly, it was in a different form, a journal, and those who were intimidated by the poem (because they were not used to discussing poetry) might find it easier to discuss this text; finally, it gives an account of the progress of the illness and includes references to drugs and medical care, and these features would establish a certain level of familiarity for the health professionals in the group.

Extract from May Sarton's *After the Stroke: A Journal*

Sunday, June 15
Will the time come when I can listen to Mozart again? What keeps me from playing records, like a finger across my mouth? The fear of a complete howling crack-up? Or that poetry would then seize me and shake me to pieces like a wild animal with prey? Who knows?

Friday, June 20
I'm entering a new phase. Monday and Tuesday were very hard days. On Monday I simply stayed in bed, feeling too sick to make the effort even of getting up. Nancy, the wise one, persuaded me to call Dr Petrovich's office and

tell one of the nurses, who said at once, 'We'll find time tomorrow for you to see the doctor,' and it was set for four-thirty. When he saw how upset I was, and close to despair because of never feeling well, he suddenly asked, 'How would you like to have the cardioversion tomorrow?' It felt like a reprieve and of course I hummed with hope and said 'Yes, by all means.'
[Cardioversion is an electric shock which often gets the heart back in sync when it has been fibrillating. Of course I was a little nervous lying on a narrow bed in Intensive Care for a half-hour or so before Dr Petrovich arrived and the machinery could be set up. Then I was alone again and by now quite tense. ... When the cardioversion finally took place I was anaesthetized for a few seconds and it was over.] Dr Petrovich said, 'It's fine. It's done the trick!' Euphoria! I was a prisoner set free. ...
But then when a nurse brought me *the* pill, Amiodoroni, the one that makes me ill, I realized I was being asked to go back to hell. It was a traumatic reversal and a storm of tears popped out of me. Late that night, around nine-thirty, after I had gone to sleep, now in a private room with the same lovely view I had had before of a line of trees against the sky, Dr Petrovich came in. Yes, I have to take the pill or have another stroke. The hardest thing psychologically to take is that he does not believe this drug makes me sick. He insisted it was the fibrillation that did. So I am on the drug, one a day for a week, then one every other day.
Dr Gilroy also came in to see me and said if I am still as miserable in two or three weeks to go and see him. This was comforting.
I woke to nausea and begged for something to help, and they did give me something which unfortunately made me very groggy all day. ...
But that night in the hospital when I lay and tried to face what must be accepted, I realized that a kind of aloneness is with me now. I have to curl up deep down inside myself. For the moment I have no energy even for the telephone. This is a new phase as I wrote at the start today – a phase in which I am more alone than ever before.
A steady downpour outside this morning matches my mood and I rather like this wild, wet world.

Monday, June 23

Again Saturday and Sunday I gave up and stayed in bed. I see clearly that the psychological problem is that I see no change – with an operation one gets better, some hard days, but the movement is there towards healing. If I had terminal cancer I would be on my way elsewhere, movement of another kind. But for five months I have been on a plateau of misery.
So something has to change and I have made an appointment with Dr Gilroy for tomorrow.

Notes: *After the Stroke*

Like the poem 'After an Operation', this extract from a journal begins with a question. Fear is also present for this person and again it has the effect of changing the person's sense of herself. Interestingly, this experience of fear also has phases. Unlike the poem, this journal documents specific events, although questions remain unanswered. Reflecting on fear is still, in this context, an uncertain process of approaching it with questions. The imagery used here is powerful – 'seize me and shake me to pieces like a wild animal with prey' – and conveys the sense that this person has of being out of control. Because this is a journal, stages in the experience of illness are well documented: 'I'm entering a new phase'. The sense of being out of control is related to this person's lack of energy to get out of bed or to seek help. Use of the passive voice emphasizes the sense this person has of not being in control: 'it was set for four-thirty' rather than 'I' or 'We set it for four-thirty'.

Aloneness is the other dominant theme in this extract; this person is left to wait alone and feels isolated in her experience. The imagery used to describe her illness again conveys her sense of lack of control, but in a different way: 'I was a prisoner set free'. At this point in the journal, moreover, it is someone else who sets her free; there is no action she can take to break free. The doctor, or the treatment, act on her for good or ill. 'Hell' is how she describes the illness, but at a point of 'traumatic reversal'. At various stages clinical decisions have been made 'suddenly', and with each decision she has a strong emotional response which takes her by surprise: 'a storm of tears popped out of me'. Her coping strategies, in this phase, include using her imagination, in visualization, focusing on externals like, for example, a 'lovely view' and socializing with a friend. None of these is effective against the distress caused by what she sees as the doctor's unwillingness to believe her description of her feelings. This low point is marked by two paragraphs which are much shorter than the others and report her experience with the minimum of detail: 'Dr Gilroy also came in to see me ... all day'.

Finally, the aloneness seems to become more acutely painful, psychologically, than she has ever felt before. Her precise problem, as she defines and feels it, is that there is no prospect of improvement in her health. She feels she is stuck at this point. This psychological effect is equally as strong as the physical effects of her illness, but here she feels she can take the initiative: 'So something has to change and I have made an appointment with Dr Gilroy for tomorrow'.

Reactions to this extract, in discussions, focus on a number of topics: the drug 'Amiodoroni', what is it for and what does it do?; the predicament of patients who have no prospect of recovery; the predicament of those who care for these people; the difficulty of dealing with psychological effects, how do we know?; that is not our job, that is for trained counsellors; the attitudes and expressions of this person – 'This is very American ... complaining so much!' This last point could be a strong prompt for discussion and reflection on assumptions and feelings among carers.

The third text, Robbie Kydd's *Auld Zimmery*, was chosen because it is different in form and content from the other two: although the narrative is still in the form of a first-hand account, it includes exchanges between characters in direct speech; although it is in the form of a short story, it also includes extracts of the main character's own journal; although his view of carers is not generally sympathetic, there is one significant exception and one significant relationship that does provide mutual comfort.

The background to this extract is that a young, punk care assistant has the same name as his late wife, Fiona. What initially seems like his confusion of two Fionas turns out to be his recovery of the memory of his wife's death:

Extract from Robbie Kydd's *Auld Zimmery*

'No, I was ...' We are quiet for a while, while I try to remember what I was going to say. Darkness, suddenly lit by a searchlight from Fiona.

'Ye've wrote it down here that yer wife deserted ye.'

'Yes, she ...' It won't come out, so I bury my face deeper in the sweet punk-scented warmth, experiencing a pain like an orgasm. I'm coming alive, I think, just let me die again.

'My boyfriend's deserted me an I'm no greetin.' So something **has** happened to her. She's in pain too. I lift my face.

'Tell me.' If she does, maybe my pain will go away.

'Naw. It's you that's greetin, stupit.'

So out it comes. The glory that was my Fiona. My plump and faithful childhood friend; my passionate spring-time lover; the mother of our two beautiful and successful children; the talented artist; the resourceful helper; the companion of our sweet autumnal re-flowering. I wax poetical and a part of my mind insists that Fiona slips right under the duvet and holds me close. But she rumbles me. She would, wouldn't she, being her.

'An efter aa that, she left ye?'

At that, it's back to where the comfort is, and more wet tears. But there's iron in Fiona as well as comfort. There always was, since our sandpit days.

'She left ye?'

I feel a kind of swaying motion. I think Fiona has picked me up in her arms and is rocking me like a baby. I wet myself warmly. You-know-who won't like that. Andy is a bad boy.

I don't know if I can write the next bit, but I must, for at last I've 'come up with something', with Fiona's help. I'm sure of it. Wet with tears as well as urine. I must pin it down on paper.

'We lived in a top floor flat.' The tremors in my voice are more than just senile. My hand trembles as I write. Fiona won't be able to read a word of this. 'A wee studio. After the children had gone. We stayed in it longer than we should have. The stairs. They were too much for me.'

'I ken aboot thae kinda stairs.'

'Fiona had to help me up and down. And carry the messages. She was always so strong. I stopped going out. One day I had to go to the doctor. When we came back she was carrying the messages. And helping me. We stopped half-way up for a rest. She fell down. Just dropped to the stone floor. She was breathing. No one answered when I rang the bells on the landing. Everyone was out at work. I shouted. No one came.'

'Aw jeeze!' She strokes my hair.

'I went down on my hands and knees. I couldn't tell if she was still breathing. I couldn't feel her heart. I couldn't move her. I started to crawl up the stairs to our own door. I was going to phone for help. I only reached half-way.'

'I cannae bear it. I'll have tae, noo. Whit happened?'

'I don't know. Next thing I was in hospital. They were dressing me up to come here. Nobody's ever told me what happened ... Nobody's ever mentioned ... Till you said ... wife ...'

greetin = weeping; ken = know; messages = shopping

Notes: *Auld Zimmery*

Although this narrative reproduces the direct speech of characters, it also gives the thoughts of one character, in the form of internal mono-logues or short 'asides' to himself. This shows the old man's reactions to events in his own terms: his spoken sentences are often left unfin-ished, but we know what he is thinking because his thoughts run on. His efforts to recover his memories and his ability, sometimes, to rec-ognize when his memory is failing him offer a contrast between appar-ent senility and lucidity: 'We are quiet for a while, while I try to remember what I was going to say ... I'm coming alive, I think, just let me die again'. His ability to read the emotions of one care assistant is ignored by other characters in the story, or perhaps they just do not see this side of him. Fiona, by contrast, does see the emotional, and sex-ual, side, and both of them see the overlap between what others in the narrative would see as very different lives. There is a comic incon-gruity in the image of Fiona, a punk care worker, complete with tat-toos, in the context of the other, more traditional care workers and their more repressive regimes. This incongruity is then modulated in the spontaneous compassion of Fiona's response to the old man: 'I cannae bear it. I'll have tae, noo. Whit happened?' Her compassion makes her much less of a comic figure.

At the end of this extract the old man discloses the details of his wife's death for the first time. He reveals how little he knows of the event and, because carers are also mentioned in his description, there is an implication that they have failed to tell him what happened. Another interpretation is that his memory has been coming and going and that he has been at this point before – apparently discov-ering and disclosing the details of his wife's death for what he thinks is the first time. But this latter interpretation is not emphasized in the story at this point. What is highlighted is the common understanding between this old man and Fiona, and the gap in understanding and sympathy, from his point of view, with other carers. There are many potential talking points in this character's representation of the care assistants.

Reading the text aloud is not something that the facilitator is required to do, nor are the participants (as this produces an interpretation of the text); instead, participants will need time to read or re-read the texts for themselves (even if readings were distributed well in advance of the meeting).

However, using the words of the text, saying individual words, lines or sentences, is important, particularly in the second half of the discussion. Initially, health professionals will be more comfortable saying medical words than literary words, and the contrast between the two may seem, at first, a bit odd – since this perceived oddness is quite revealing in itself, it can be the basis of an interesting discussion. In other words, the newness and oddness of some aspects of these discussions can make interesting subjects for discussion. These discussions often reveal the different assumptions and expectations – both about medical humanities and about their own professional practice – within the group.

The discussion will, if well structured, produce a mixture of views, and it might be as well not to have made your mind up at the start. Even if you cannot think of any lines for discussion, or if the ones suggested in this chapter do not turn up, you can still use the strategies for developing ideas, including the writing activities, to make sure that people have time and means to develop their own ideas. Once they have raised a point, interaction can be encouraged. Referring participants back to the text and encouraging closer scrutiny of individual words is the facilitator's next task.

Variety

This selection of texts was, therefore, intended to provide variety, in the forms used, the background of the writers, the approach taken to the subject and the representation of the medical or caring environment.

Variety of texts is equally important for promoting wide-ranging discussion. This has been a principle of our text selection in our group. The aim has been not to allow any one frame of reference to dominate our discussion – neither the frame of reference of any one text nor of any one participant, including the facilitator.

Cycle of reflection

The general pattern of each discussion is a cycle of observation and reflection: participants

- **express their own observations** on the text;
- are then prompted to **express a view on a specific question**;
- discussion then allows for **comparison of views**;
- and the final stage is **further reflection** on our initial observations, with **initial views consolidated or modified**.

Timing

Over a 1-hour session the timing for these four phases is as follows: 10 minutes for introduction and expressing individual views (and perhaps more, if reading time is needed); 10 minutes for writing and pair-sharing; 30 minutes for plenary discussion; and 10 minutes for final reflections. If the session is to run for 2 hours – as ours do – these timings can be doubled:

1.	Introduction (and reading) – expressing individual observations	10 min
2.	Expressing a view on a specific question	10 min
3.	Comparing views	30 min
4.	Consolidating or modifying initial views	10 min

These timings indicate the proportions of time allocated to each phase in the discussion. This general pattern has proved effective in initiating and sustaining discussions in our group over the past 5 years. The role of writing activities, as the mechanism both for expressing individual views and responses to specific questions, has been critical in this process and this will be dealt with in more detail in this chapter.

Open questions

Open questions can be used to prompt discussion, even when the nature of the discussion is completely new. For example:

'After an Operation': what kind of experience does it present?
How would you sum up this person's feelings?
What is your gut reaction to this poem?

What is your reaction to the person in the journal *After the Stroke*?
Do you get the feeling that she is working through her problems well?
What do you think of the care she is receiving?

What image of the elderly is presented in *Auld Zimmery*?
Do you like or dislike the main character?
What did you think of the use of direct speech?

It is important that the questions at this stage do not have a literary frame of reference, so as not to be off-putting. The vocabulary of literary criticism or the frame of reference of the linguistic analyst can be quite intimidating. Without it, participants can be prompted to react to the poem in their own terms and in their own words. The aim of the discussion is not to reveal the 'right' answer but to prompt many different answers. The role of the facilitator is to encourage participants to reveal their own response – any response – to what they have read. In fact, the variety of interpretations is important; it stimulates and challenges further reflection. It also adds an element of surprise: we can never predict what people will say, though we can be sure of one thing – that we will not all agree in our interpretations.

Some of these questions, therefore, deliberately invite participants to draw on their own experience and to make their own subjective judgements. This is an important first stage; if participants do not achieve this, if they do not make their own judgements, then it is likely that they will revert to trying to find the 'right' answer. This is why the questions are directed explicitly at the participants, with consistent use of 'you,' as in 'What do you think?' 'What is your reaction?' and 'Do you like or dislike?' in order to direct the participants to focus on their own views.

Focusing questions

A focusing question can prompt debate. For example, a good question for prompting discussion of the poem, 'After an Operation,' is:

Has this person fully recovered?

This question deliberately avoids the word 'patient', as in 'Has this patient fully recovered?' Definition of the word 'recovered' is left to the individual reader. This question picks up on the ambiguity of the last line, 'Yet I am not the same': is this 'not the same' positive or negative?

Similarly, a focusing question for *After the Stroke* would likewise focus on a particular word or phrase in the text, for example:

> What is keeping this person on a 'plateau of misery'?

This question requires readers to move beyond their own impression of the character to the character's impression of herself. This is an important distinction in this text and part of the character's problem with the quality of her care; i.e. she is distressed by the difference between her image of her illness and her carers' image of it.

Auld Zimmery, finally, is finely balanced between comedy and tragedy and a focusing question would be one that encouraged participants to focus on this balance and to decide for themselves which way it tips at certain points in the narrative. More importantly, they can be encouraged to shift their attention from their initial observations and judgement, the critical first step, to the frame of reference of the characters: i.e. does the old man **see himself** as comic or tragic? Useful focusing questions could be:

> In what way is Fiona, the care assistant, like a 'searchlight'?
> How has she managed to have this effect?

The open text

Most literary texts, it can be safely assumed, are open to more than one interpretation. The facilitator can form questions from those words or phrases which have more than one interpretation. This sometimes opens up the whole text, questioning interpretations of other words in the text, which can then be seen to have more than one meaning. Moreover, in discussion participants bring out these differences, rather than moving towards a group consensus. Sometimes additional questions are raised by the group and, rather than stick with a fixed agenda of questions, it is often much more rewarding to move on and discuss these.

Again, these questions are designed to stimulate debate and therefore must be open, perhaps general, perhaps allowing for ambiguity in interpretation but certainly having more than one answer. Facilitators aiming to design their own questions could use mine simply as models for their own, in the first instance. Alternatively, they could listen to questions that emerge from group discussions.

If we can assume that a literary text has many possible interpretations then we should expect that any group of readers will produce these differences. Even readers who are not experienced in interpreting literary texts can form a judgement and/or personal response to a first-hand account, particularly if the group is medical and the subject is familiar in its medical context.

Writing about the texts

Writing tasks are a key element here. They give participants an opportunity to voice their views. Short, private writing activities of 5 minutes in response to an open or focused question work to prompt the individual response. This writing then forms the basis for the individual's contribution to 'pair-share' discussions. This prepares participants to have something to say in a plenary discussion.

The 5-minute writing tasks developed for this context are based on the technique of freewriting developed by Peter Elbow (1973, 1981). It is a technique that has proved successful in helping people to overcome writing blocks and develop writing skills. Pure freewriting is an activity that is 'free' from both audience and purpose, two of the strongest influences on our writing. Freewriting is not addressed to a reader and is not intended to achieve a specific outcome.

Freewriting has been adapted for the medical humanities context: writing for 5 minutes; without stopping; in sentences; not correcting grammar, punctuation, spelling; not for a reader. Writing in this way is, according to participants, liberating: they do not worry about what someone else will think about their writing and they do not stop to edit what they write. Those who find the idea of freewriting odd, and those who prefer to plan before they write, are simply invited to see this activity as trying something new. This short writing activity is used at several points in all our discussions.

As an initial activity freewriting provides material for the pair-share and then plenary discussions. At the end of the session it allows participants to express their views and then compare their final writing with their first. It is seen by participants in our group as a surprisingly productive and enjoyable activity, giving people time to reflect, to make up their minds, to sort through their thoughts and, sometimes, to find out what they think. Some participants enjoy the peace that descends on our group as we write.

Over time, people have begun to share their writings, but at least one of the writing activities is designed to be private, in order to allow that liberating effect to take place. The choice of allowing someone to read the writing, or not, is always left to the individual.

How do you get people to say anything?

A good starting point is to ask questions that invite subjective answers and opinions, using the words 'In your opinion ...?' This can produce quite opinionated discussion but it is a start, and it will almost certainly provoke a response in other members of the group.

Writing activities, particularly if they are to be kept private, allow people to develop their own views in their own way, at their own pace and in their own terms. This can prepare them to have something to say.

Sooner or later someone will begin to talk about their experience, which may take the discussion far away from the topic of the text but will, again, prompt others to respond by drawing on their experience.

A key technique here is to encourage participants to respond to each other, to play one contribution round the group, as and when people choose to respond. This may mean leaving a momentary silence while people think about what they want to say. Above all, the facilitator must, in the early stages, take a back seat.

Basic group management and participation skills come in useful here. The key principles in the preceding paragraphs will be obvious to those with experience in this kind of teaching or management. These principles are briefly outlined here because they are crucial to the success of early discussions in a medical humanities group.

Patience and tolerance are useful qualities, given that some participants will challenge the use of this kind of discussion and the frame of reference of some of the questions. Others will see meanings of words as fixed, in medical contexts, rather than fluid, in a variety of personal contexts:

What's the meaning of 'convalescent'? – That's obvious!

The response here has to be, 'OK, let's see how we do define it'. In other words, if this statement is opened up to the whole group it should produce some variation across the group. If not, then that too can be a talking point. Alternatively, at a later stage in the discussion, the group could explore what the person in the poem takes this word to mean. Thinking about the meaning of words in context is the point here: this word has been used by a particular person in a particular context and we ought therefore to reflect on their particular view of the meaning of the word. It may be that other words used by the person, in the context of the text, may provide clues to their use of the word. The context can also shape our interpretation as we read, but our reading is often complicated by our bringing in, naturally enough, our own context.

Some participants will question the purpose of analysing a literary text:

> Aren't we overanalysing here?

Again, there is no need for the facilitator to come up with 'the answer' to this question; the group can produce a variety of answers and the facilitator's role is rather to bring these out. This question can be an interesting talking point: at what point did the discussion move into 'overanalysing'?

Some participants feel a bit lost in the variety of interpretations:

> Surely the writer didn't intend all these interpretations!

The writer's intentions are difficult to establish, even for the writer. However, the question of what is the range of reasonable interpretations, for any one text, is interesting: at what point do we feel that we have strayed too widely in our interpretation? What are the elements that seem to take it beyond what is in the poem? And why is this a bad thing?

Finally, there are those who seek to educate the non-medical members of the group, aiming to explain the literary text by explaining the medical subject:

> What you have to understand, Rowena, is that in a hospital ...

This is fair enough. Participants are to be encouraged to draw on their own experiences. Furthermore, this kind of response will also prompt responses from colleagues in the health professions, who will have varying experiences and may challenge a statement that is over-generalized, where the speaker has assumed that the statement is universally true.

Medical terms can produce a certain reaction among participants: 'This word only has one meaning', 'In a medical context that word can only mean ...', or 'You can't start interpreting medical terminology in your own way'. These statements, often strongly put, reveal a challenge to the fixed and factual vocabulary of medical discourse and discussion. The question raised here is whether medical terms are fixed, with only one meaning, or open to interpretation and judgement. This question can take the debate away from the literary text and towards individuals' use of language in their professional lives, an interesting tangent which can have participants comparing their assumptions about specialist languages.

This is where pointing out that the point of view is not medical can be helpful in reminding participants that they are not reading a medical report, from a medical point of view, but a first-hand account of a patient. So the question 'What does convalescent mean?' might have only one medical answer; but the question 'What does convalescent seem to mean to this person?' prompts us to check precisely how the word has been used in this poem. Does this word have the purely medical, or dictionary, definition in this person's point of view? After all the expressions of 'fear' and 'dread' in the first and second verses, does 'convalescent' really convey the sense that the person feels she is recovering? Why is it the only word – apart from 'operation' – which is drawn from the medical context? Which context(s) are the other words drawn from?

In other words, participants have first to be encouraged to say what they think. Later they can be encouraged to focus on the precise context of the writing, the precise associations of the words and the point of view of the writing, which will always shape our interpretations of the words.

What people said about 'After an Operation'

Has this person fully recovered?

What do you mean by 'recovered'?
She's still preoccupied if she's writing about it.
I wonder what kind of operation she had?
I wish we could look at her chart.
Obviously she has recovered. There's a new strength there.
Obviously she has not recovered. There's a sense of loss at the end of the poem.
Well, she's recovered physically – it says 'convalescent' – but not psychologically.
What makes us think this person is female?
Why did no one tell her what to expect?
This poem made me realize I did not fully prepare a patient yesterday for her operation.
How can we tell which patients feel this way and which don't?

We don't have time to talk to the patients.
But does **the patient** think she's recovered?
What does 'convalescent' mean to her? To me it means ... but to
her it seems to mean ....
I had a patient like this once.

How to get people to develop their interpretations

As discussion progresses the focus can be shifted to the poem by questions about particular words or phrases. This usually has the effect of prompting participants to develop or modify their interpretations. For example:

Prompts for developing interpretations

Why does the poem start with a question?
Why does *After a Stroke* start with five questions?
What effect does this have on our reading?
What kind of 'first impression' does it establish of the character?
What is the effect of the use of 'I' in the first verse of the poem?
What is its effect in *Auld Zimmery*, paragraph beginning 'I went down on my hands'?
What happens to that first person in the second verse of the poem?
What is the effect of using it so often in the first verse and then hardly at all till the end?
The character in *After a Stroke* uses the word 'alone' often; what makes her feel this?
In *Auld Zimmery*, why does the old man confuse the two Fionas? Did you find this convincing?

These questions can prompt participants to re-read carefully certain lines. Therefore, reading time and time for all participants to find the relevant section of the text may be required. They can then check their own interpretations and process each other's.

What roles is the facilitator playing?

The facilitator can work to validate the variety of languages which people use in discussing the poem. Literary and non-literary languages are taken to be equally valid. This is particularly true if the facilitator is known to be trained or expert in literary criticism, or even if they are known to have a literary background. This will require the facilitator who does have a literary training to modify his/her own language for discussing the poem, although it must be said that this facilitator has to take a back seat in early discussions. Their role at this early stage – and perhaps for some time – is to encourage others to speak up and to develop their confidence, and their vocabulary, in talking about literary texts.

The facilitator

Non-directive
Not being the 'funnel' for all comments
Structuring and shaping
Leaving, or creating, open phases
Chair
Introduce
Encourage

Organize tea/coffee etc.

Observe

Spot who is ready to talk

Organize the reading, writing, speaking activities
Select or organize (and distribute?) readings
Provide questions for discussion
Provide prompts for closer study of the text

'Challenge' categorical statements with neutrality

Conclusion

For the participant: Be ready for the challenge of differences of view.
    For the facilitator: Be ready for questions, but do not feel you have to answer all of them.

Summary

- **Reading time**: Everyone reads the poem individually (instead of giving a reading, aloud, which would probably influence people's interpretations).

- **Getting started**: Discussion can be started quickly with one question – 'Has this person fully recovered?'
- **Thinking time**: Then there is time to decide, individually, on their own answer to the question.
- **Writing time**: They are asked to write this down, giving reasons for their answer. These reasons must be based on the text, so they are asked to refer to specific words in the poem.
- **'Pair-share'**: The next step is to compare responses and reasons with a partner.
- **Group discussion**: This is a plenary discussion, in which participants reveal a rich diversity of interpretation, frequently surprising each other with the range of views from the same text.
- **Writing time**: Each person does a short piece of writing that sums up their own answer to the question.

6 The next step: *Blue Above the Chimneys*

Something for everyone ● Targeting interests in the group ● Initial reflection ● Encouraging talk about the text ● Discussion ● Shifting the focus of discussion back to the text ● Looking for links and gaps between your view and what the text says ● Drawing out different views and different interpretations ● Further reflection ● Literary observations

As the group establishes itself and grows more comfortable and relaxed, participants will find that it is safe enough to tackle even taboo areas of health and personal and professional relations. In this chapter I will follow through the 'next step' for the group in a discussion of difficult issues and in the learning experience of the group.

The above list of issues will be covered in this chapter within the framework of this discussion. The purpose of this chapter is, above all, to show the structure of the session, dealing with the issues in context. By working through three texts, this chapter offers guidelines for guiding a group's discussion. The extracts were chosen for discussion because they represent experiences of illness and the effects of illness on those who are close to the patient: lovers, family and friends.

Although the subject matter of each text is illness and distress and the treatment of this subject is very moving in each case, our discussions of these texts have been stimulating and even enjoyable. The process of engaging with these texts, writing about them and discussing views and issues with others has surprised some participants; they have been surprised to find that such unhappy subjects could provoke such stimulating discussions.

Continuing with the format outlined in previous chapters, this chapter proposes three phases for discussing each text: initial reflection, discussion and further reflection. Extracts of the texts we have used are included here, along with suggested lines of discussion. The framework for our discussion was defined in previous chapters in general terms and is illustrated here in specific terms. This involves some repetition of the outline framework in this chapter, repetition having the function here of recap and reminder.

The session starts with an introduction by the facilitator: welcome and introductions, brief definition of medical humanities (for new participants), choice of texts and outline programme for this session:

Programme

Introductions (10 min)
Medical humanities (5 min)
Texts: introduction (5 min)
Texts: reading, writing, talking (1 h 30 min) + Break (10 min)

---

1. *Blue Above the Chimneys*, a novel by Christine Marion Fraser: Initial reflection, discussion, further reflection
2. *Elegies*, poems by Douglas Dunn: Initial reflection, discussion, further reflection
3. *Cancer in Two Voices: Living in an Unstable Body*, a journal by B. Rosenblum and *Cancer in Two Voices: Living in My Changing Body*, a journal by S. Butler: Initial reflection, discussion, further reflection

The priority at the start of the session is to help people to feel comfortable in the group. There is, of course, a variety of techniques for achieving this and there seems no reason why they should not work in this context. Clarifying names and roles is helpful. Repeating introductions over several meetings can be useful, as new people join the group. The facilitator can clarify his/her role as guide and/or chair in the discussions.

There is usually a certain amount of paper shuffling at this stage, as people sort through their readings and outline programme or gather up copies of readings if they have not received them in advance. The facilitator can check that everyone has copies of the readings, knows the loose agenda and has a cup of tea or coffee to keep them going (if need be).

The choice of texts for this session shows variety in terms of subject, point of view, background of the author and form of writing. Fraser's novel was chosen for accessibility – it is a narrative which is easy to read. Dunn's poem was chosen not only because of the force and immediacy of his descriptions of grief, but also because we aim to include poetry in all of our sessions. Rosenblum's and Butler's narratives were chosen because they present two views of cancer – the view of the sufferer and the view of the partner. This selection therefore includes male and female writers, heterosexual and lesbian relation-ships, points of view of sufferer and partner, prose narrative and poet-ry, novel and journal, and adult's and child's points of view.

As I illustrated in the previous chapters, our discussions have been structured around three activities:

- Initial reflection
- Discussion of questions
- Further reflection.

To recap: this is the general framework for our discussion. Suggestions for each of these stages are provided for each of the three texts in this chapter. There are also suggestions for writing – private writing – which can provide material for the discussion at each stage. This writing can be shared, or not, during discussion with a partner and/or in the plenary with the whole group. One session lasts about 2 hours. Three readings may be too much for one 2-hour session or it may be just right; it depends on how the discussion goes. Texts that have not been discussed can be held over for future sessions.

Ideally participants will have had time to read the texts before the meeting but since this is sometimes impossible there is usually some demand for reading time at the start of the session. Selecting one text for this first reading stage – for example Christine Marion Fraser's *Blue Above the Chimneys* – can speed up this process. Those who have already read the text often find it useful to do some rereading at this time.

Fifteen minutes' reading is not wasted time; those who have read and perhaps re-read the first text for discussion can move on to read-ing the other texts. This is often a time when people begin to make a few notes.

Extract from Christine Marion Fraser's *Blue Above the Chimneys*

The summer smells filtered faintly in through the windows but it wasn't enough for me. I wanted to embrace the sky, to roll on the earth, to feel the whip of the wind tugging my hair. I pined for the bitter-sweet familiarity of family life. Beds were objects to be hated. I thought if I ever got out of hospital I would never want to sleep in a bed again.

Never having been a child for gazing into mirrors, I wasn't aware of my changed appearance till one day I got a glimpse of myself in the long mirror of the physiotherapy department, which I attended twice a week for wax baths and exercise. At first I didn't recognize myself and stood staring solemnly at a thin little sprite with a white face. My hair cascaded in auburn waves down my back to my waist. The nurses were forever admiring it and brushing it but I had never even bothered to look at it. Seeing its beauty I no longer wanted Kirsty's bobbed locks. I stared at myself, feeling I was looking at a stranger, a cruel shadow who was mocking me because the frail shell of my body had, by a chance in a million, contracted a rare disease for which there was no known cure.

After spending nine weary months in hospital I was sent home. It was Christmas time and the wards sparkled with trees and tinsel. Now that the long-awaited departure from my cocooned world had arrived, I felt oddly apprehensive. Vaguely I remembered the grey tenements of home. In comparison, the hospital seemed suddenly bright and gay. The trees, sparkling with a thousand lights, were a big attraction to a little girl who had known only home-made decorations strung across a dingy room.

Secretly I knew I was clinging to straws. I knew that life consisted of so much more than superficial things like Christmas trees and tinsel. I had grown up a lot in hospital. It was difficult to remain a child in a world of life and death, pain and boredom. My quick restless spirit had been stifled in an existence that demanded a great deal of patience.

So I went home. The doctors could do nothing for me except wait for the next stage of my illness to show itself.

It was strange and frightening coming home to the tenements. Grey chimneys loomed into grey skies. The streets looked dirty after the clean white world of hospital. Suddenly I dreaded meeting my brothers and sisters again. I who had been the leader in mischievous games now felt an intruder into a world that had become foreign to me.

I arrived at the close in an ambulance and children who had once been my playmates stared at me with the blank, round-eyed detachment of strangers. They were gathered in a tight curious knot near the ambulance, snot-nosed, grimy faced, giggling, whispering, all belonging to each other and shutting me out.

As I walked slowly out of the ambulance and into the close I realized that my life would never be quite the same again. The thought came swiftly into my brain. At ten years and nine months old I felt adult, wise and very sad.

pp. 85–87

Initial reflection

This initial activity aims to give participants a chance to reflect on their own views about this story. In private writing, writing that will not be shared, there is an opportunity for free reflection. The writing is short – only 5 minutes. It is important to stress at this point, as participants often view the first writing task with some trepidation, that the writing need not have any structure – any beginning, middle or end – and that grammar, punctuation, spelling and any aspect of style are not important in this writing. The writers can also move about from topic to topic, following a train of thought or jumping from one idea to another. The writing should, however, be in sentences, not in note form, without getting bogged down in what exactly constitutes a sentence.

Reactions to writing this may vary: some find it immediately, or ulti-mately, liberating to write without an audience; some enjoy having time to express their own thoughts and feelings in this way; others find the task strange and unusual, unlike any other kind of writing they do; some are put off because they think that the writing has no purpose. This latter group can be put off by the apparent failure of this 'freewriting' to achieve quality: 'What's the point of doing bad writ-ing?' one postgraduate student asked me recently. Encouragement is therefore sometimes essential: encouragement, that is, to see freewrit-ing not as 'bad writing' but as a chance for the writers freely to articu-late their own views, thoughts and feelings. Once people start writing, we have found, this activity almost always becomes a thoughtful and peaceful 5 minutes.

A prompt for writing can be simply:

> What is your reaction to this child's description of her return home?

This can encourage an immediate response to the description, leav-ing the writer free to choose the focus; this question does not impose any particular issue or focus on the discussion. This kind of question often produces two kinds of response: one which sees in this narrative the pattern for long-term patients generally and another which focus-es on the specifics of this child's experiences. Both responses – and oth-ers – have a place in the discussion. In fact, the variety of responses is one of the most stimulating effects; we can never anticipate partici-pants' responses and we have learned not to expect to achieve con-sensus. This makes anticipating the responses of a group, which is part of the point of this part of this chapter, quite difficult. What I am doing here, therefore, is sketching patterns of our discussions, in our group, in the hope that this provides possibilities for new groups and a safe-ty net for new facilitators.

Once people have started writing it is often difficult to get them to stop. It is not crucial to stop after exactly 5 minutes, but more than 10 minutes might become a bit like hard work and might lose the spon-taneity, moving towards a developed interpretation rather than an instant impression.

Once everyone has stopped writing, perhaps with encouragement (to stop) from the facilitator, then there can be a 'pair-share' session, where participants discuss their views, revealing as much or as little of their writing to each other as they choose, since the writing was intended to be private. They are, of course, free to choose to let their partner read their writing (with no pressure on the partner to reciprocate). And these guidelines can be offered explicitly and briefly to participants as they move from writing to talking.

The discussion is usually lively, as both people (in the pairs) can go into their own and their partner's views in some depth. After 10 or 15 minutes, depending on how discussion appears to be going, the facilitator can move the discussion on to the plenary discussion.

Discussion

This is where the full range of observations opens up, as participants draw on their initial reflections, their personal and their professional experience to articulate their interpretations of the text.

Discussion of *Blue Above the Chimneys* will probably touch on long-term patients, institutionalization and the process of readapting to home life. There is usually some interest in the medical condition itself and in the physiotherapy context. If the extract does not include enough detail on this, then some background and context could be provided by the facilitator or by anyone who has read the whole book. But this is not essential, since even a short literary text can provoke a wide range of responses.

A general statement on the main topic, touching on one or two issues is often enough to get the discussion rolling. For example:

General introduction: summary

The topic of this extract seems to be the child's perceptions: her view of hospital, of herself and of her home and family. Her mixture of emotions, from anticipation to apprehension, at the prospect of going home are described from her point of view. Her description reveals the gap which has opened up between her hospital life and her home life, between her hospital self and her home self, just at the moment when she is realizing this for herself. In fact, this is the moment when she literally sees the change for herself when she looks in the mirror.

This kind of general statement – summing up the main points – can help to focus the discussion on the text. The statement is part summary and part interpretation. Other participants may have other versions of the summary and this can also spark discussion. The summary sometimes seems to bring participants 'back' from their own narratives, if they have wandered away from the text, although my feeling is that going off at tangents is not wrong; alongside our tangents the literary text continues to prompt reflection. Furthermore, reflections on experience –personal and professional – can be interesting to other members of the group and there are no boundaries for balancing observations on the text and stories from experience that have been triggered by the text.

Boundaries do, however, seem to have evolved in our group: the most personal of experiences are explored more in the pairs than in the plenary. In other words, allowing time for private writing and pair-sharing may be providing a safe, limited forum for personal discussions, thus filtering them out of the plenary discussions.

Wherever the discussion roams, however, the facilitator can bring the discussion back to the text. As participants' attention returns to the text there often emerge comparisons, implicit and explicit, between people's interpretations and what the text actually says. However, if participants themselves do not see this at first, or at all, the facilitator is under no obligation to point it out; others in the group may do so, or the realization may take place later in the discussion, or some time afterwards. The facilitator may or may not see him/herself as responsible for shaping participants' learning outcomes. In our post-qualification, non-assessed, mixed group, participants have been free to develop their own 'outcomes'. In a more formal educational context perhaps the facilitator would take a more directive role, although readers' experiences, however limited, would surely still have an important place in this kind of reflective discussion.

The extent to which readers' experiences shape their interpretations is, in any case, an interesting talking point and one that could be an interesting subject for further reflection in the final writing task in this session. This 'shaping' effect is often clearer after discussion and re-reading of the initial writing, produced at the start of this session. 'Correcting' readers' interpretations is not, I would argue, the priority here. At this early stage in the group's work, as they are beginning to feel comfortable with literary texts, using the discussion time to generate a broad range of responses rather than a limited range of appropriate interpretations is the priority.

Medical subjects, therefore, do not always dominate the discussion, since there are numerous references in the extracts to personal perspectives on the medical conditions. Even the health professionals in the group find themselves differing in their interpretations and this, again, is part of the point: to open up discussion to dialogue rather than diagnosis, to interpretation rather than investigation, to emerging commentary rather than clinical conversation. As health professionals develop a level of ease and expertise – usually quickly – with a literary text and with dialogue, the unlikeliness of agreement in interpretations becomes the spark.

This range of interpretations can be provoked by individual words. For example, 'cocooned' (p. 86) implies a safe place, but it has both positive and negative connotations. Discussion of people's interpretations should probably, at some point, include a definition of the **meaning** of the word: the case which houses a growing creature, the silk worm. Then there are its **associations**, the different meanings we associate with the word, in different contexts: protectiveness and nurturing. Yet 'cocooned' can also suggest a stifling effect. It is unlikely that all participants will attach all these meanings and associations to this word. Discussions will draw all these out. Then participants can consider which they feel predominates, in this context, in their reading of this text: the safety or the suffocation?

Safety and suffocation both feature in this chapter of the novel in the meanings and associations of other words in this extract. There is the safety of the hospital, yet it also has a stifling effect on the child's development. Ironically, her home offers a similar conflict for her – the 'bitter-sweet familiarity of family life' (p. 86) is also a 'world which had become foreign' (p. 87).

So which impression predominates for each reader? In reflecting on this question there will be some discussion of personal views and experiences on the process of institutionalization. There could be further discussion of the word 'cocooned' itself, of other contexts in which it has been used or read, for example.

'The meaning of this word is obvious' is a view that comes up from time to time, as a participant begins to feel that we are making too much of one word. Here the facilitator can validate the process of looking for variety in interpretation and illustrate this, by summing up the range of views in the group. Alternatively, this could be an opportunity to explore further the process of 'making too much of one word', to look more closely at the implicit or explicit critique. Some participants may prefer to discuss the process of considering meanings and associations in such detail. There will be a certain novelty for some in the idea that a single word, even a medical term, can have more than one meaning, and certainly more than one association, to other members of the group and even to other health professionals. It may be worth pointing out that the group has not selected every word for detailed discussion and that some have found their attention has been drawn to the same word, which raises another question:

> What is it, then, about the word 'cocooned' that has attracted this kind of attention?

Some participants will simply be fascinated that so much can come from one word, in one short extract.

Someone may question the process of discussing literary characters in this way as if they were real people. This is also an interesting point and it can help to spend time considering the differences between discussion of real people and discussion of literary characters: there are interesting differences in both content and form. The discussion of literary characters has opened up possibilities that might not be appropriate in discussion of real people (particularly among those who are responsible for treating the people). This may be a good time to explore feelings, apprehensions and prejudices about discussing literary texts.

Context is the key in interpreting words: for the word 'cocooned':

Is there a context for either of the 'safety or suffocation' interpretations?

Are there other words in this extract that suggest that 'cocooned' should be read more as safety than suffocation?

These questions led us to the observation that both interpretations were there, both appeared to feature in this context, both seemed present in the point of view of the main character. Both were there for the character and therefore had influenced the word choice. Both were part of her story, her version of events. This raises the question of what the child was aware of and what the adult narrator adds to the account.

Point of view shapes the telling of the story and also shapes our reading. This story is told by an adult recalling her experience as a child, filtered through the (fictional or autobiographical) memory of the adult. Without overcomplicating things here, it is worth thinking about the question of point of view:

Who is telling the story?

What perspective do they have on events?

Can we, the readers, gain any insight into how this perspective has been constructed or influenced by events or by other people?

How do we account for our answers to these question by referring to the text?

Again, some people will see these questions as obvious and will anticipate some equally obvious answers. However, while there may be some general agreement on general answers, there will be variations and each person will articulate their answer in their own language, using their own frame of reference.

The next step: *Blue Above the Chimneys*

Another possible way to develop this phase of discussion is to invite questions from the group:

> What other words or phrases have caught the attention of other readers in the group?

Participants may have different focal points, perhaps coming out of their initial reflective writings. Some readers will have latched on to the meanings and associations of other words. Exploration of these words could follow, along the lines of my discussion of 'cocooned'. The words they choose may also turn out to be connected to the contra-dictory associations of 'cocooned'.

In the discussion that now follows I will attempt to sketch in some possible directions for the discussion, based on my own reading of the text and on my observations of our group.

From the very start of this extract (p. 85) the child appears to want to be active, to break out, rather than be 'cocooned': 'I wanted to embrace the sky, to roll on the earth, to feel the whip of the wind tug-ging my hair' (pp. 85–86). These words suggest that she wants to get out into the elements and to feel them physically. The hospital repre-sents, at this point, a place of confinement. By contrast, the next para-graph describes her sudden awareness of her physical changes during the 9 months in hospital. Her body now seems to her like a 'frail shell' (p. 86). This shell image is not unlike the cocoon image; both are designed to protect the inhabitant and in some way their purpose is to protect creatures while they are developing. The irony for this child is that, while hospital has been perceived as a place of recovery, she is returning home with the illness and its effects. Even though she will no longer be confined in the hospital she will continue to be confined within her body. The language used here suggests that the child's image of herself is of confinement, with a possibility of a change in, though not freedom from, her disease.

The next paragraph clearly defines her ambivalence towards going home. Her fear colours the images of hospital and home, making their contrast visible to the child: 'Vaguely I remembered the grey tene-ments of home. In comparison, the hospital seemed suddenly bright and gay' (p. 86). The use of 'vaguely' here reveals the sketchiness of the child's memory which, after 9 months, is swamped by her fears.

The idea of growth – in a cocoon – is further developed in the next paragraph: 'I had **grown up a lot** in the hospital. It was difficult to remain a child in a world of life and death, pain and boredom' (p. 86). However, the idea of suffocation – in a cocoon – is also developed here:

'My quick restless spirit had been **stifled** in an existence that demand-ed a great deal of patience' (p. 86).

Both resignation and determination are conveyed at the end of the chapter in one short sentence: her matter-of-fact 'So I went home' could convey both the child's spirit, which helps her to move on to the next phase in her life, and her resignation at her own and her doctors' inability to change her condition. Her spirit is threatened on her return home because her familiar role in the family appears to her to have changed. Her growth in the family context has been stunted: 'I who had been the leader ... now felt like an intruder' (p. 87). Some readers may interpret this change as, in itself, a kind of growth and there could be a very interesting discussion which attempts to recover the child's sense of her own position:

> Does she see herself as growing and nurtured or as stifled and stunted?

She calculates the effect of the changes for herself as she leaves the 'cocoon' of the ambulance, seeing herself as growing a further step away from her former self: 'I realized that my life would never be quite the same again.... At ten years and nine months old I felt adult, wise, and very sad' (p. 87).

The final image, in this extract, shows her leaving her cocoon both physically, as she returns to her home, and emotionally, as she acknowledges that she cannot be like the other children, or perhaps like the child she once was.

The role of the facilitator can be very much in the background of this discussion, perhaps even separate from the discussion, allowing participants to generate their own observations without going through the 'filter' of a group leader. During early meetings, however, a group may look to the facilitator as a marker of the appropriateness of individual interpretations and it is useful to have strategies for deflecting the kind of eye contact that can make the facilitator literally the focal point of a discussion. New participants in an established group may have the same reaction, looking to the facilitator to endorse or reject individual responses. If the facilitator is a literary expert – in any sense – then this reaction can be strengthened by participants' sense of their group leader as the person to judge the value of contri-butions and they may expect comment before they feel discussion can progress. Again, this in itself could be a talking point, a prompt for an airing of expectations.

If the facilitator is not a health professional – in any sense – participants may attempt to educate him/her about the 'real' medical context and the 'correct' interpretation of a text about a medical subject. For example, a participant may focus on 'wax baths and exercise' (p. 86) and discuss the nature and timing of these treatments in some detail. An interest in the medical condition may make participants curious to know the exact history of the disease (in the previous 85 pages of the novel), its diagnosis and its treatment. They may then choose to educate the facilitator on the appropriateness of the child's treatment and care. This is something for the facilitator to deal with: it may be the participant's expression of resistance to a particular interpretation; it may be a covert invitation to endorse or reject an interpretation; or it may be the beginning of a thinking-out-loud process. Whatever the motive, this apparently didactic approach may be frustrating for the facilitator and opening up the discussion to include other participants is usually effective in deflecting confrontation and defusing frustration.

To sum up, this section has defined some of the ideas and issues raised by this extract. The method for encouraging discussion consists of simply starting with participants' observations initially, and then focusing on some detail in the text. In this case, this was a matter of starting with one word which had evoked a strong response: the word 'cocooned'. If this word has been identified by members of the group, as often happens, then so much the better.

These notes have, to some extent, followed the pattern of a discussion, as readers probe the text, 'testing' it against their interpretations, introducing narratives of their own experience, forming different kinds of observations and judgements about the narrative and about the discussion itself, and sharing opinions and information.

This extract from the novel is not a case study and it has not been discussed as if it were. The main point has been to open up discussion to include personal and professional views, as well as assumptions and attitudes, as well as emotional and intellectual responses. Initially this means giving people an opportunity to articulate their own view privately. Then the discussion demonstrates that the range of reactions can be very broad indeed.

Further reflection

After the discussion there can be time for further reflection, using writing again, this time in order to consolidate or modify an initial reflection. The writing task can take exactly the same form as the initial writing task:

- 5 minutes' writing;
- unplanned and unstructured;

- with no concern for continuity, for grammar, punctuation, spelling or style;
- in sentences rather than in note form.

This writing can be either private or for sharing, with the facilitator and/or the group or individuals deciding. Participants can work with the same pair-share partner or choose or be allocated someone else for the discussion after the writing. The facilitator can be useful here in clarifying and reminding participants of the proposed form(s) for writing and discussion before people start to write.

The prompt for reflective writing at this stage – should one be needed or requested – could simply be to compare views expressed in initial writings with views expressed in the group discussion:

> How do participants respond to the text at this stage?
> How does this view compare with their own earlier view?
> Do they have any new points to mull over?
> Do they want to return to the issue that interested them earlier?
> Have they consolidated or modified their earlier view?

The next reading is from a collection of poems about the death of the poet's wife from cancer. Douglas Dunn's *Elegies* chart the diagnosis, the stages of her illness and the stages in his grieving. The poem 'Second Opinion' focuses on the moment when he realizes that the first diagnosis was correct. Most of the poem's six verses are about his reaction to this realization. The person with the illness is hardly mentioned at all in this poem (although she is mentioned in many other poems in this collection). In fact, details of the cancer and its effects on the patient are not included at this stage; the impact of the cancer on the partner is the main point here. (Again, these general, summing up points could be used as a prompt for initial writing or for the plenary discussion.)

Second Opinion

We went to Leeds for a second opinion.
After her name was called,
I waited among the apparently well
And those with bandaged eyes and dark spectacles.
A heavy mother shuffled with bad feet
And a stick, a pad over one eye,
Leaving her children warned in their seats.
The minutes went by like a winter.

They called me in. What moment worse
Than that young doctor trying to explain?

'It's large and growing.' 'What is?' 'Malignancy.'
'Why **there**? She's an artist!'

He shrugged and said, 'Nobody knows.'
He warned me it might spread. 'Spread?'
My body ached to suffer like her twin
And touch the cure with lips and healing sesames.

No image, no straw to support me – nothing
To hear or see. No leaves rustling in sunlight.
Only the mind sliding against events
And the antiseptic whiff of destiny.

Professional anxiety
His hand on my shoulder
Showing me to the door, a scent of soap,
Medical fingers, and his wedding ring.

Douglas Dunn, *Elegies*

Initial reflection

As with the previous text, initial reflection on this poem could be prompted by a general question, perhaps enquiring about the reactions of this person to the news:

How would you describe the effect the news has on this person?

While the answer to this question might seem quite obvious to some readers, the initial reflection (5 minutes' writing) and pair-share will inevitably produce both common ground and differences across the group, and perhaps even within the pairs.

The primary aim of this question is to stimulate writing and discussion, and therefore it will not hurt to make an easy start with a general question, though it might make matters clearer if the facilitator says so, in order to reveal the purpose of the question and the point of the writing. It might also be helpful to make explicit the expectation that the writing and pair-share will produce different answers to the apparently obvious question. Furthermore, as participants begin to answer the question the facilitator can encourage them to provide references to the poem to support their readings. This is usually more challenging and should provide further discussion about shades of meaning and interpretation of individual words, phrases and images.

For example, here is one answer to the question, which readers could compare with their own; i.e. readers could write for 5 minutes –

now – then read the example below and in this way gain some insight into the range of interpretations that can be stimulated by one short text and one general question:

One reader's answer to the question (5 minutes' writing)

I think he's just beginning to face up to reality, heading into shock, plus envying the doctor with, he presumes, his healthy wife and denial and fear at the prospect of the cancer spreading. This all amounts to a mixture of emotions for this man, although I notice that there are few explicit references to his emotions. But he does reveal fear and anxiety in what he says to the doctor and in how he says it. So what is my overall answer to the question? – the effect the news is having on this person is that he finds himself isolated by the news: 'No image, no straw to support me' suggests that he feels that he has to cope without support. He does not feel any support from the doctor, whom he sees as off-hand, in 'shrugged', and as putting on a professional mask, in 'Professional anxiety' and relying on routine, in 'Showing me the door'. As the doctor distances himself emotionally, professionally, from the case and from this man's emotions, he ends up in a kind of void – 'nothing/ To hear or see'. Overall, he seems isolated or alienated by the news and since his partner is absent from the poem, perhaps this is his first appreciation of separateness, or separation, from her?

This writer has constructed an answer to the question in the course of writing; i.e. this writing was not produced from a plan or outline. It drifts away from the question at one point and returns to it in the second half. The writer then attempts to pull this collection of observations together for an 'overall' answer to the question. The links with the text are also there, supporting one interpretation, and in fact these quotations seem to push the writer towards an interpretation. Perhaps the last line takes this writing beyond the question, but the writer has made an interesting observation in the process: it is noticeable that the person experiencing the illness is absent.

This writing activity – writing for 5 minutes, in this way, even on a simple or general question – does in practice produce stimulating variations and food for thought and discussion. The lack of strict boundaries for, and the privacy of, the writing allow members of the group to digress and raise further questions for debate.

In comparing this 5 minutes' writing with a partner and with others in discussion, there will inevitably be differences and overlaps:

- Some may have paid more attention to, and written more about, the **narrative** in the poem, i.e. the progression from waiting and watching (verses 1 and 2), to talking and reacting (verses 3 and 4), to thinking, imagining and leaving (verses 5 and 6).
- Others may have focused on the **role**, or the **image of the role, of the doctor** presented here.
- The arresting use of direct speech, in verses 3 and 4, will probably have attracted attention and comments.

At this stage – discussing initial reflections – the aim is to open up the poem to a wide range of observations and initial interpretations by the group, with as many people contributing as possible (and with the facilitator taking a back seat, apart from encouraging everyone to have their say).

Discussion

As we saw with *Blue Above the Chimneys*, a more focused question could prompt further discussion:

What are the implications of the word 'shrugged' in line 13?

Answers to this question will vary: some will reply that it conveys the callousness of the doctor; it conveys the apparent lack of emotion; it conveys the perception of the partner that the doctor cannot possibly share his feelings at this point. Placed as it is after the line which most strongly conveys personal anxiety – 'Why **there**? She's an artist!' – the word 'shrugged' strikes a strong contrast, suggesting lack of emotion by comparison. While the patient's partner is distraught and angry the doctor appears, to him, distant and off-hand. Some in the group will see this as 'professionalism', as the professional's ability to stand back and not get overinvolved: 'Professional anxiety' is one of the poem's observations on the doctor's behaviour.

Again, while this question seems to be straightforward and while we might all expect to have roughly the same answer, in practice the subtle differences and perhaps not-so-subtle assumptions and expectations that we have built up to justify our actions and support our interpretations become rich material for debate. So the question is, in fact, quite debatable, but it is often after people begin to contribute their answers that the discussion really takes off. People can then see the variations for themselves. In fact, it is often quite surprising how many different interpretations and reactions a literary text can stimulate.

Further reflection

Since participants had less to say about this poem than about the other texts, this stage of further reflection was particularly important, in order to give each person time to develop their own views. A prompt for further reflective writing could be to invite participants to go back to their first 5 minutes' writing:

Do you have a 'second opinion' on this poem?

This could be an opportunity to develop an initial view in a number of ways:

- to change your mind
- to elaborate on your first opinion of the poem
- to write about a related topic
- to write about some aspect of the poem related to your work.

These are suggestions for reflective writing, intended to leave writers free to choose their own focus or to develop one in the course of writing. These suggestions might be helpful during early meetings. However, in practice, we have found that participants have done so much talking and listening by this stage that they have plenty to think about and may not need any specific topic or direction for their reflective writing. This may vary, depending on the make-up of the group, in terms of age, experience, education, work, etc.

Links between the two readings can be a topic for writing, whether or not they have come up in the discussion; a summary of specific issues which have come up in discussions of both 'Second Opinion' and *Blue Above the Chimneys* can be used here as a further prompt for reflective writing:

Did you notice any links between 'Second Opinion' and *Blue Above the Chimneys*? Do you see any similarities in the characters' responses to incurable disease?

What images of carers, of treatments and of the hospital environment are represented in these two texts?

Blue Above the Chimneys is a first-hand account and 'Second Opinion' is the point of view of an observer. How has the point of view affected the presentation of the medical subject and emotional reactions?

Suggestions for reflective writing are there to be used by those who need them and to be ignored by those who do not, and this point is worth discussing with the group.

Moreover, the main point of reflective writing is that it should come from the individual's thinking at this stage, rather than from a prompt from the facilitator. This is why the questions above use the word 'you', so as to encourage an individual answer. This is also why the example of the 5 minutes' writing exercise used the word 'I', to show personal point of view. Writing in the first person – using 'I' – may be completely new to many participants, except for personal letter writing, and it may be useful to allow some time for discussion of views on this.

Perhaps the facilitator should allow time for re-reading of initial writings (before or after this reflective writing). Some groups can, of course, be directed to, or may request that they can, structure their own time in this final phase of the discussion of this text.

The lack of prescriptive instructions for facilitators in this section is quite deliberate. What is provided here is a starting point: suggestions for activities and generalizations about how groups have tended to react to these suggestions. If all of these suggestions are offered to the group then people will be free to choose. If, however, the facilitator 'reads' the group and sees that people are looking for more structure, then there is a case for directing even the reflective writing.

Facilitators can feel free to try out a range of possibilities or to offer possibilities and note which ones people take up and use. This flexibility can also be shared with the group; the facilitator can discuss possible writing activities, for example, or give a personal view on one or two, inviting others to do likewise. This could lead to a negotiation about preferred activities for talking and writing. Variety is important, however, and with the agreement of the group the facilitator is there to vary the texts and activities to prevent routine setting in.

The facilitator's participation, or not, in the writing and talking activities is worth thinking about and perhaps discussing with the group:

Should the facilitator take a back seat throughout the session, in order not to provide too strong a steer to the discussion?
Should the facilitator do the writing tasks?
Should the 'back-seat' facilitator find something else to do while pairs and groups are talking, so as not to seem to be eavesdropping?
Should the facilitator be a non-participant observer, taking time and making space to observe and respond to the reactions of the group?

Joining in the writing activities can help to make them seem less like a 'test', which participants have to do but facilitators do not, and can make facilitators aware, first-hand, of the participants' point of view in discussions of the writing tasks. The answers to these questions may be quite individual and a certain amount of 'playing it by ear' will help the group and the facilitator to develop.

Extract from Barbara Rosenblum's *Cancer in Two Voices: Living in an Unstable Body*

My doctor put it to me very clearly: I had to have chemotherapy, surgery, and radiation, in that order. I had to have chemotherapy for three months before surgery because the tumour in my breast was too large to remove surgically. It had grown too quickly and was now virtually inoperable. Chemotherapy would shrink the tumour, permitting surgery without skin graft. There was another reason for chemotherapy first: the cancer had spread to my lymph nodes, including a supraclavicular node near my collarbone. That was an indicator that metastatic processes were already occurring throughout my body. It was a serious, aggressive cancer and I would require the most aggressive treatment available.

Before the first treatment, my doctor prepared me for the various side effects I might experience. My hair would fall out, I'd have mouth sores, I'd vomit, and I'd lose my period. So, after the first treatment, I vomited about thirty times in forty-eight hours, had tired muscles and aching joints, and was exhausted from spasmodic vomiting. Even if you didn't have cancer and just vomited that much from a flu, you'd be exhausted. And that was just the first week.

The second week, I had low blood counts, extreme fatigue, and breathlessness from the lack of sufficient haemoglobin – and consequently oxygen – in my blood. Almost exactly on the twenty-first day following the first set of three injections, my hair began to fall out. Not just on my head. I lost my pubic hair as well. But I still had my period.

After the second treatment, I had all the side effects again. And I still had my period. I thought for sure I'd beat this: I wouldn't go into menopause.

Following the third treatment, I had all the same side effects but, this time, I had a shorter period. Still, I didn't attend to it much because, by this time, my nose and anus were bleeding from chemotherapy and I grew alarmed. It seemed like I was bleeding from new places and losing the familiar bleeding from familiar places.

Barrington, J. (ed.) *An Intimate Wilderness: Lesbian Writers on Sexuality*, Eighth Mountain, Portland, OR, pp. 133–134

Extract from Sandra Butler's *Cancer in Two Voices: Living in My Changing Body*

I begin writing this sitting at the kitchen table drinking tea and listening to the eager clacking of her typing. Barbara has just begun to write a piece about her body, her changing relationship to it and has announced quite firmly that she wants to write alone. I sit and chafe, wishing we could work together, wondering what she will write about our sex life, our changing intimacies. Wanting to be included. Last week I spoke at the Women's Building about sexuality in the relationship of a couple dealing with life-threatening illness. It was very well received, and many of the women seemed relieved to hear me verbalize what they were experiencing in physical or emotional isolation. I was both moved and grateful for the response, and it deepened my conviction that the writing Barbara and I are doing is vital in the lives of other couples living through many of the same struggles.

I spoke to them about our sex life, how it used to be, how it is now, how we have accommodated the physical changes in her body, the emotional changes in her psyche, and the relational changes in our daily lives. I didn't talk like that, though. I talked in daily language. One of need and dependency. Mostly mine. Of an inwardness and sometimes excruciating thoughtfulness. Mostly hers. I talked about the way I was socialized to be an appropriate heterosexual and had lived for nearly thirty-five years in response to the sexual needs of others and how hard I struggled against that early conditioning when I came out as a lesbian. I spoke of how easily I find myself slipping back into those old roles again. How I find myself feeling that Barbara's needs are the real needs and mine are not. That her feelings are the ones that matter, and mine don't. That the frequency, the form, the intensity of the sexual dimension of our lives will – no, should – be determined by her. Not by me, and rarely by us. Just like it was before, when I was in my twenties and thirties. Actually, I know it isn't like before, but I do admit to an uneasy similarity sometimes.

Now I sit here wishing she would call to me from her office down the hall and ask me what I would add to this piece. What is it like for me, as her partner? How does it feel to have lived for eight years with a woman who now has advanced cancer spreading through her body?

Barrington, J. (ed.) *An Intimate Wilderness: Lesbian Writers on Sexuality*, Eighth Mountain, Portland, OR, pp. 139–140

Initial reflection

A starting point for initial reflection could be writing for 2½ minutes on each of the texts, in answer to an open, non-threatening question. This is particularly important here because some readers will be more preoccupied with the description of sexuality than others; in this case, it is important to enable participants to find their own starting points:

What is your overall impression of each narrative?

This would produce two shorter pieces of writing, a variation on the 5 minutes' writings, also inviting comparison and contrast of the two texts, or of the two voices or of their two responses to the same cancer. If getting started with this writing proves difficult at first, participants can use the words of the question to prompt their writing: i.e. 'My overall impression is ...'

Follow-up questions can be used to help participants to develop their ideas:

> What are the markers for this impression in the text?
> What words suggest this impression to you?

Such questions may have become familiar to participants now. The facilitator will have asked these questions often enough, and participants can have a look at their own writing to judge for themselves. They could then pinpoint one or two words in the text which have shaped their first impressions.

Examples of 2½ minutes' writings are provided here in order to illustrate what one person produced in this way. Again, readers can try doing their own writing first and then comparing it with the writings below, to get some of the effect of doing the pair-share:

On Rosenblum (2½ minutes' writing)

My overall impression is of someone focused on her illness and finding a creative way out of it, but still caught up in it. It's like a learning process – learning the science, the symptoms, her changing body. The word in her title, 'unstable,' does come through in the writing, but she seems stable.

On Butler (2½ minutes' writing)

My overall impression of this is of someone whose life has become consumed by her partner's, understandable, especially if she feels guilt as well as love. I worry about how she will manage when Barbara dies. She has 'changed' in parallel and in the direction of Barbara. (Is this also inevitably 'unstable' although she hasn't used the word?)

Follow-up questions could be, for example:

> What are the markers for these interpretations in the texts?
> What words suggest these interpretations to you?

The facilitator often asks these questions in discussion, but participants can take another 5 minutes to have a look for themselves at their own writing. They could pinpoint one or two words in the texts which have shaped their first impressions, perhaps focusing on the opening sentences. This could be an idea which they see appearing, perhaps in more than one form, more than once in the text. For example, Barbara Rosenblum's writing gave one writer the impression of 'learning', and on closer inspection it does include a list of learning points, showing the evidence of instruction by her doctor in words like 'virtually inoperable', 'indication', 'supraclavicular node', and 'metastatic processes' (p. 133); while in the second half she is balancing this against her own experience and in her own language, such as 'bleeding from new places'. Similarly, in Sandra Butler's writing one writer's first impression was of a person consumed by her partner's cancer, and this is clear from the very first line, where she is simultaneously writing and listening to her partner writing, 'wishing we could work together' (p. 139). She also describes other activities that centre on her partner and her cancer, although these activities do also allow her to include her own experience as the partner of the person with cancer. That her life has been rearranged around her partner is most clearly indicated later on this first page: 'How I find myself feeling that Barbara's needs are the real needs and mine are not. That her feelings are the ones that matter, and mine don't' (p. 139).

Discussion

Our discussion of the whole extract included in the anthology, of which the extract used here is a part, moved participants in our group by the description of these people's love for each other. Some participants also expressed their concern for Sandra Butler, because, they felt, she seemed to be putting her own life too much 'on hold' and appeared to be suffering in her own way in the process. That this was her reaction to her partner's cancer, her way of expressing complete and unconditional support, was a view that was also put forward, but the balance was judged by most to have tipped from sympathy to selflessness in a negative sense. It was also acknowledged that this person has a right to express the impact of her partner's cancer on her life and that it might benefit her to do so.

Ironically, this mingling of the two stories in the two writings seemed to have the effect of confusing the identities of the two writers in our discussion, to the extent that people found it difficult to remember who was who. The distinctions were blurred from the start by the similarity in the titles: *Living in My Changing Body* and *Living in an Unstable Body*. One pair of participants took the unusual – in the sense that no-one else in the group did this – step of referring to one of the writers as 'she' and to the other as 'he'. This was seen by some in the group to be a disturbing subversion of the identity of one of the women and of their relationship. Others made no comment on this. Clearly, the subject of lesbian sexuality will challenge some readers more than others. Some were comfortable discussing this. Some made no comment on it. Some used the word 'lesbian', some did not. Some later said that they had felt uncomfortable in this discussion.

No additional questions were needed to progress discussion of these two readings. Everyone had something to say about the relationship and the way the two people were dealing with the cancer. The interaction between the two texts seemed to provide a rich variety of contrasts and comparisons. This kept people thinking and talking. 'Encouraging talk' was, in this case, a matter of encouraging talk about the specifics of the two writings. For example, if someone commented that there is often suppressed anger, for partners and patients, the facilitator could ask, at some point, whether there is evidence of this in these writings: i.e. whether this is reading between the lines, or drawing on personal or professional experience, or picking up on the emotional content in the writings.

Those who had a professional interest in the subject – working in oncology – were able to contribute background information, knowledge and personal views about the process of caring for and supporting cancer patients. Those who worked in cardiac rehabilitation contributed parallel examples to illustrate the effect of serious illness on the patient's partner. The positive power of involving the partner in rehabilitation was discussed. The complications – for example, exclusion – of gay and lesbian partners were explored. The emotional, not just the medical, course of an illness became part of our discussion, since it features so strongly here.

The patient's point of view, once again, was seen as offering essential insights into the processes of being ill and being treated. The possibility of an active role for the patient was favoured, qualified by discussions of feasibility, resources, staffing and time. 'Wanting to be included' clearly voices this need, although there was some discussion about how much influence the health professionals could have in this context, since it is in the writing, rather than in the caring, that the partner wants to be included. There also seems to be a sense of exclusion: 'What is it like for me, as her partner? How does it feel to have lived for eight years with a woman who has advanced cancer spreading through her body?' (p. 140), which some also felt conveyed anger. Others saw this as less a matter of suppressed anger and more a matter of expressed grief, since she is writing and expressing her feelings here.

Suppression of her – Sandra Butler's – identity came up again and again in this discussion. Her link between the 'shadow role' she was playing with her partner and the subservient role she saw herself as having played as a heterosexual prompted some discussion of the roles women in particular may play in this situation.

Both writers reveal their struggles to express what they are feeling and these writings, while revealing the difficulties and barriers, can be seen to be taking these struggles further forward; i.e. in writing they seem to be sifting through the issues and 'translating' the illness into their own terms. This use of 'writing to yourself' or 'writing for yourself' was compared to the short private writings produced in this group, with participants describing their enjoyment of the writing and their surprise at this enjoyment.

The use of different languages is also important to both writers. The ending of the extract from Barbara Rosenblum's writing is less medical, more personal, replacing medical English with everyday language: 'bleeding from new places and losing the familiar bleeding from familiar places' (p. 134). This contrasts quite strikingly with the first sentences, with its rational and clinical explanations, where cause and effect are clearly defined: 'My doctor put it to me **very clearly**: I had to have ... **in that order** ... **because** the tumour was ...' (p. 133). The use of different languages, technical and non-technical, is also important to Sandra Butler, who translates her experience into plain English: 'I didn't talk like that, though. I talked in a daily language' (p. 139). This again raised interesting questions about communicating with patients and partners and also about enabling people to talk or write about their emotional reactions. There were also reservations here among those who felt that this was not their territory, or not their area of expertise. Some said they would feel out of their depth.

The patient's predicament is revealed, in Barbara Rosenblum's writing, as not knowing how much or how little to make of their symptoms and changes in the symptoms. These changes trigger for her the expression of instability, highlighted in her title for this writing. Her observations – 'Almost **exactly** on the **twenty-first** day following the **first** set of **three** injections, my hair began to fall out' – plots the illness and treatment in detail and with clarity but paradoxically cannot, for her, make it any more stable. So many influences – social, sexual, medical, physical – are destablized.

Further reflection

The last stage of discussion, possibly after another 5 minutes of reflective writing, is a quick exchange of views in pairs or in plenary.

Closure in discussions can be a problem, particularly if, as often happens, time is running out. However, in practice, in our group, there has been no great desire to achieve closure. Besides, the facilitator cannot know whether or not participants have found their own form of closure, since the facilitator will not have seen the private writings nor heard the final pair-share discussions.

Looking back on the discussions and showing consensus and openness can, therefore, be a useful rounding off strategy here:

- Participants themselves can form collective, individual or group conclusions.
- The facilitator can summarize the discussion and make a contribution.
- Non-participative facilitators may have observed movements in the discussion or issues which were not dealt with or which are still open to debate in the group.
- Without forcing a consensus the facilitator can pull together the work of individuals' and group discussion at various stages throughout the session and highlight the collective efforts, the dialogues and the breadth of the discussion.

Themes and connections which have emerged, or have not, in the discussion can be underlined here: the impact of illness on the partner; identifying with the sufferer; the power of institutionalization, and institutional roles; the use of narrative to bridge the gap between medical explanations and first-hand experience of illness and treatments.

Finally, participants can be encouraged to say whether or not they have enjoyed the session. Since most will have found it stimulating, this discussion could take some time. It seems important, in our group, that the discussions are not only interesting for professional reasons, or 'uses', but also to register personal enjoyment. Participants have recorded in feedback questionnaires that they enjoy our medical humanities group because it is for themselves.

Vocabulary for talking about literature

Initially this should not be an issue: in the early stages any vocabulary will do. At some point participants may seek to use the language of literary criticism, but the option to use any language at all should remain open.

For those who have felt unsure of some of the terms used in this chapter and do not feel that they themselves can use them yet, here are some definitions:

- **Point of view**:
- Who is telling the story?
- How have they shaped the story?

- Is the story told from a particular position?
- *e.g. an adult? a child? a medic? a bereaved partner?*
- **Verse**: A group of lines in a poem ('stanza' is an alternative)
- *e.g. Dunn's poem has six verses*
- **Style:**
- Look at the way things are expressed, the tone, the language used, look at individual words and sentences
- *e.g. medical and plain English in Butler and Rosenblum*
- **Meaning:**
- The sense of a word, or the intended sense
- There is more than one meaning for each word
- What a word means in practice
- What a word means in context
- *e.g. meanings of the word 'grief'*
- **Associations:**
- Links we make between ideas
- Links we make between words
- *e.g. linking 'cocooned' and safety or suffocation*

7 Taking a theme: *The Trick is to Keep Breathing*

Different texts on the same issue – death and bereavement • Initial reflection and questions – encouraging 'puzzling' over a poem • Discussion and comparisons between texts • Further reflection • Summary • Extending this discussion

---

> ### Texts

1. 'The Door of Water', a poem by George Mackay Brown
2. *All in the End is Harvest: An Anthology for Those Who Grieve*, edited by A. Whitaker
3. *The Trick is to Keep Breathing*, a novel by Janice Galloway

This chapter illustrates the theme approach, taking the subject of death, as dealt with in different texts in different ways and forms. Unlike discussions that dealt with several subjects, this focus allowed wide-ranging and in-depth discussion of one subject. The theme approach described in Chapter 4 is therefore illustrated here in much more detail. Timings for part of this discussion – for the third text – are given as a guide for facilitators.

Each of the selected texts tackles the subject of death in a particular way: George Mackay Brown's poem starts by encouraging us to 'think of death' and to meditate on its forms and 'meaning'; the extract from *All in the End is Harvest* looks at one of the most famous poems about death, Dylan Thomas's 'Do Not Go Gentle Into That Good Night', which seems to encourage us to confront death as aggressively as possible; and Janice Galloway's *The Trick is to Keep Breathing* describes the painful process of dealing with the death of someone close, particularly when the grieving process has no social context.

This chapter uses the framework established in previous chapters for structuring discussion: initial reflection, discussion and further reflection. What is different about this chapter is that the first part is built on questions raised by the group. This is because our first text raised so many questions that this outcome in itself had to be addressed in our discussions. In fact, I used this string of questions to encourage people not to be put off by what they did not immediately understand on their first or subsequent readings.

I was also trying to get the group to generate their own answers, however partial or tentative they felt them to be. Those who lacked confidence in dealing with poetry could be reassured by the discovery that the poem had raised similar questions for other readers. This reassurance could then enable them to begin to answer their own and others' questions. This progressive questioning also illustrated the process of puzzling through a poem, working with the more complex and compact (than prose) structure and the varieties of word use that often appear in poetry.

Initial reflection and questions

The poem we chose was George Mackay Brown's 'The Door of Water', which opens with an invitation to 'think of' death. It was these 12 lines that prompted an unexpected, and to some participants incredible, range of interpretations. Perhaps the poem's approach to the subject of death helped to produce this range of readings for us; because the poem consists of clearly distinguished sides of, or 'doors' to, death a number of different responses were triggered by each door; each door opened up a range of interpretations for the readers.

The Door of Water

> Think of death, how it has many doors.
> A child enters the Dove Door
> And leaves a small wonderment behind.
> For airmen there is the Door of Fire.
> Most of us, with inadequate heart or lung or artery,
> Disappear through the simple Door of the Skull.
> There is the Door of the Sheaf (the granary is beyond).
> The very old enter, stooping,
> Harvesters under a load of tranquil sorrows.
> For islanders, the Door of Water.
> Beyond a lintel carved with beautiful names
> The sea yields to the bone, at last, its meaning.
>
> George Mackay Brown

Perhaps it is because this is not a narrative poem – a poem with a story – that it raised many more questions for our group. Without a story line it was more difficult to follow the poem's 'train of thought'. It was difficult to hold all the lines and all the images of death together. In fact, it required some thought, some 'puzzling', to work out what particular lines and half-lines of the poem meant and what the whole added up to.

The group and individuals could, it seemed, progress without answers to some of their questions. As facilitator, or literary expert, I avoided taking responsibility for answering these questions and used them instead to structure and progress discussion gradually. This was partly because I wanted participants to explore their questions for themselves and to find out for themselves that this could be a productive way of working with a literary text, and partly because, as I freely admitted, I did not have all the answers to their questions. In this way the questions did not become a stumbling block to discussion, but were instead seen as a prompt for definition, clarification and reflection – as food for thought for the literary expert as much as for the participants. Questions became a reason to stop and think.

This variety of questions could also be seen as a feature of the variety of participants; i.e. this was not a dialogue among medics, or among nurses or among physiotherapists. In fact, not all of the participants worked in medical or related fields. This range of participants could be another factor that prevented any one treatment of the poem from dominating the discussion.

What follows is an account of this process: the questions raised by participants and the many and varied answers they produced. In case this process of questioning seems intimidating or mechanical, I should add that when asked if she remembered our group's discussion of this poem, one participant enthusiastically said that she did, adding emphatically: 'Yes! I thought that was one of the best nights'. Some participants in our group found this a very emotional poem; what appeared, at first, to be abstractions and apparently factual statements about the subject paradoxically, on further readings and analysis, created a very emotional effect for some.

At the start of this session, participants had very little to go on in the way of background on either the poem or the poet. Some had heard of George Mackay Brown and knew that he was a writer from Orkney, a writer who had, in fact, spent very little of his life outside Orkney and had written mainly about Orkney in his short stories, novels, plays and poetry. Many had heard of his novel *Greenvoe*, which has recently been included in the Scottish secondary school English syllabus. Some knew that I had written a PhD thesis on George Mackay Brown's prose, but I kept this quiet on this occasion. So most read the poem very much out of context, particularly since there are not many references for context in the poem.

Filling in the background to poems was attempted by readers who took the content to be autobiographical; in other words, they assumed that this poem includes 'airmen' (line 4) because George Mackay Brown was possibly/probably in the RAF. That this is far from Mackay Brown's experience (one of the few factual details I provided) made it easier to see the risk in reading literary texts as if they were the writer's own voice or thoughts. This was a useful reminder to us not to read literary texts as if they were documents from the writers' lives. If the literary text is creative, then the chances are that the text will express ideas which interest the writer, but it is a fallacy to say that authors even intend all of the interpretations we make of their texts. And even if a writer were to have certain intentions, these might not appear in our interpretations. We spent a little time discussing this in terms of this specific example – the 'airmen' – so that the issue did not become too abstract.

These questions and issues had to be dealt with before the 5 minutes' initial reflective writing. This was therefore delayed; we had by this stage become quite flexible about the timing of this writing activity. Whenever there are initial questions or immediate reactions then, we feel, these should be addressed rather than repressed.

Once the group has had this initial discussion, or if the group has been meeting for some time, then an open invitation to write for 5 minutes on the poem might be all participants need to get them started. If they do request a prompt for writing, one possibility could be:

> What is your response to the idea of death as doors ... or to particular deaths in this poem being represented as particular kinds of door?

These two questions should allow both a general response to the idea in the poem and a particular focus on a specific image, according to the interests of the individual participant.

Another prompt for initial reflection, in 5 minutes' private writing, could focus on this opening instruction to the reader:

> Did you follow the instruction to 'think of death'?

Further possibilities for initial reflection are presented in the images of death which follow the first line, reflection on the different deaths represented for different people.

Alternatively, participants could use this writing time to explore one particular image in the poem that caught their attention. Some participants may want to focus their writing on a particular death of someone they knew. This option of personal writing is always open to participants. Sometimes it is revealed in discussion; sometimes it remains private, presumably ... I say 'presumably', because I never see what participants write.

In practice, with a group of people who have been meeting for several months, I would offer both 'open time' for 'open writing', as well as prompts for writing, without waiting to be asked. This should, I feel, allow participants to pick up on the option that appeals more strongly. The basic principle I am trying to operate here is to provide something for everyone.

The initial writing can follow the routine established in previous chapters, with pair-share to follow. If the group has been writing and talking about their writing in this way for some time, then they may have developed some confidence in their ability to write for 5 minutes. They may also have developed a sense of the worth of their own views. New participants may need some support, encouragement and clear instructions or prompts if they are at different stages in this process.

Privacy is, I would argue, still an important feature of this writing stage. Individuals can, of course, choose to show their writing to their partner, but there is no obligation to reciprocate. Even a well established group may appreciate reminders, and periodic reviews, of the agreed ground rules from time to time.

Discussion

Given that the topic is death the facilitator may have to exercise some sensitivity in those phases in the discussion where his/her role is to steer the discussion away from personal experience and back to the text, while still accommodating personal experience.

Since this is not a therapeutic group, some boundaries have to be established and the facilitator may be responsible for maintaining them. Having the text as the focal point of the discussion is very helpful here, making it easier to shift focus, more covertly than overtly, in discussions. One way of doing this is simply to pose another question about the text and since there are plenty of questions in this section, facilitators have plenty of possibilities.

The private writing allows participants an outlet for personal responses; the pair-share allows more intimate sharing of feelings than the plenary discussion. Participants can use each of these different forms of expression as they wish, setting their own limits on what they reveal at each stage. Boundaries are explicitly set by the facilitator, who plays the role of drawing discussion back to the text. This is not to say that the personal experience and emotional responses are to be excluded; quite the reverse has been true in our group sometimes, as has been illustrated by summaries of our discussions in these chapters. The point is that, as we have developed our group, we have avoided developing therapy sessions, though some participants have reported that they find medical humanities a stimulating antidote to the world of work.

Limits and boundaries can be set, negotiated and renegotiated as the group develops. Perhaps imposing them from the start would have an inhibiting effect. To a certain extent the group, once working collaboratively, can adjust and assert limits in the course of any one discussion: i.e. individuals – not just the facilitator – can support and respond to each other's needs in ways they think appropriate.

This session, which began with questions, continued in the same vein: questions which had come up in participants' writing or in the pairs work were offered by participants in the plenary. These were often illustrated by references to conversations which had taken place in the pairs. Answers to their questions then began to be developed in the group discussion. The role of the facilitator was to provide reassurance, as the list of questions grew longer and remained unanswered. The questions raised are listed here, along with examples of comments and answers developed by the group.

Making it explicit that one of the purposes of discussion is to share and work on questions together is useful as part of the reassurance process. Identifying questions, finally, can be seen as simply another way of focusing on part of the text by choosing some word or line that has caught the reader's attention. Some of the 'questions' are in fact tentative answers.

Why, in the poem 'The Door of Water', does the death of a child produce only 'a small wonderment'? Would the death of a child not produce the deepest and most powerful emotions? Why has this kind of death been described in this way? Is this part of the poem conveying the poignant sense of the dead child's smallness, its unlived life? Or is this suggesting that the dead child leaves behind it a presence, in our memory of it, or as a kind of ghost? The 'Dove Door' suggests that the death of the child is peaceful. This might convey a religious conviction, if the belief is that a child dies in innocence and therefore returns to God. Is this therefore representing a religious context for the whole poem? **Do any of the other doors in the poem suggest a framework of religious faith?**

The child's death creates an arresting image in this poem, since the death of a child is very difficult to cope with. Focusing on a particular death could also direct our attention away from our own death, from any death we were prompted to think of by the first line, 'Think of death', or from any other thought prompted by this line. The word 'enters', rather than 'exits', for example, immediately caught the attention of some readers, suggesting to them a kind of ceremony. This word is slightly more formal than 'comes in'. 'Small wonderment' also suggests religious awe rather than raw emotions. We also noted that this formal language contrasts with the informality of the first line, 'Think of death'. The capital letters in 'Dove Door' also suggest a formalizing of this entrance and the capital letters are used throughout the poem to give each death its own title: 'Dove Door', 'Door of Fire', 'Door of the Skull', 'Door of the Sheaf', Door of Water'.

The participants' questions, therefore, prompted tentative observations on how language was used in the poem. In sharing observations participants were encouraged to consider their own questions further, if they felt that they were still unanswered. The facilitator can be helpful here in returning to the person who put the question in order to find out whether or not they feel that their question has been answered, and to see if others agree. Other participants also began to generate observations without getting hung up on whether or not they were answering the questions.

Our group also began to generate ideas, to piece together an interpretation of parts of the poem, not so much line by line as question by question, observation by observation, with no clear picture of the poem's meaning emerging at this stage.

We disagreed about whether or not the first door conveys a religious faith, taking the sting out of death with a vision of a spiritual afterlife. The idea of going to another destination is suggested by the words 'entered' and 'door'.

The next door in this poem is for 'airmen', whose particular kind of death takes place in the element of fire.

Why include airmen? Why not work through the various stages from childhood to old age, with a door for each, or in some other progression? What's the connection with airmen? Was George Mackay Brown, the author, an airman? Is this scene from his own life? We do not have much to go on here, because this is a very short sentence – only one line. The use of 'there is' makes it sound quite factual, suggesting that these are facts, rather than imaginings. Again, this factual style seemed to us to be the antithesis of an emotional response to the event, death by fire. We initially felt that emotions and pain were not included in the definition of this death-door.

In puzzling over this inclusion of airmen one participant in our group suggested that this Door of Fire was there to make up the four elements. The other three are all there: earth (sheaf, granary), air (airman, dove), water (water). **Why would the poet choose to include the four elements? Or rather, what is the effect of his having done so?**

The first of these questions might have led us on a wild goose chase by prompting us to attempt to read the writer's mind. The second question was more useful: it prompted us to reflect on the meaning and associations of the words used; i.e. we could deal with what we actually had: the words of the poem and our own reactions to them. We could also begin to look at the link – or gap – between the two. Questions that focus on the effect of a particular word or form are useful both for opening up interpretations and for establishing where our interpretations come from in the text. By contrast, trying to work out the writer's intentions is very difficult, though often tempting.

Tracking a writer's intentions is perhaps just another strategy readers resort to in order to explain or justify their own interpretations. The risk here is that we stray too far from the text into speculation about intentions, which cannot always be verified anyway, even by checking with the author. Alternatively, if readers are often wanting to track writers' intentions then maybe there is something in this process of 'recovering' writers' intentions. Maybe it can be another way of 'unpacking' the poem and its potential meanings. What, really, is the so-called 'risk' in speculating in this way? Even if there is a risk of misreading the poem, this does not seem to prevent readers from putting the text in their own context, or rather in a context they construct for the text. Readers will still make interpretations that do not fall within any established range of 'intentions'.

Perhaps it is important to spend some time discussing the patterns of readings that have emerged in the group. This could be a private writing activity, which might make it less threatening. Specifically, if this pattern of reading the literary text as autobiography has come up then this could be a topic for writing or discussion.

What do participants think about the idea that there is such a thing as a range of acceptable or appropriate interpretations? Literary theorists would tell us that there is a limit to interpretations of a literary text, but is this relevant to the medical humanities process, where the frame of reference is in many ways more open? These questions about ways of reading, about setting limits to interpretations and about deciding what is relevant and appropriate could be interesting topics for discussion:

Is it appropriate or useful to consider an author's intentions?
What is the outcome of this consideration?
What kind of interpretation does it produce?
What are the author's intentions in this poem?

This last question is a prompt to reconstruct the author's intentions from a reading of the poem, to explore fully the possibilities and then consider the **outcome**: has this kind of 'reading-of-intentions' produced any new insights, or any different insights? Was the **process** of this reconstruction interesting or revealing in any way? Has it, in fact, revealed something of our readers' assumptions or expectations?

However we choose to read and analyse, the text can remain the focal point of the discussion. But we cannot stop our own imaginations working. We cannot simply stop making links between the poem and our own personal experience. The relationship between reader and text, therefore, can be quite dynamic, i.e. not static. The reader need not be a passive recipient of the text. Moreover, if the aim of medical humanities is to prompt discussion, then enabling readers to interact with texts is the point, not correcting the ways in which they make these interactions. Readers will, in any case, interact differently – from each other – with texts and it is these differences, as has already been established in this book, that stimulate our open discussion.

The notion of the 'appropriateness' of a reader's interpretation, therefore, begs the question 'appropriate to whom?' Readers, in this context, have much more freedom to make up their own minds about what seems appropriate to themselves and to each other. The question of whether or not their own readings make sense in terms of what the poem actually says is one which they can begin to answer for themselves. The processes of negotiating a range of meanings and validating different meanings are perhaps topics not suited to the early stages in a group but worth focusing on later, particularly once patterns of readings have set in and perhaps threaten to 'routinize' the discussions.

These issues are potentially relevant to the discussion of a poem which does, in fact, prompt the reader to 'think', bringing the reader into an active role. Starting with the word 'think' and working through to 'meaning', the poem develops a model for thinking about death, which seems to move the reader from thought to understanding. The question is: **Has it had this effect on the readers in the group?** Some participants in our group found this a very emotional poem; the abstractions and factual treatment created a very emotional effect.

Further questions about word choice and the nature and order of the images of death were raised in our group: **Why put 'most of us' – i.e. the most common kind of death for most kinds of people – in the middle of the poem?** Why not build up to this at the very end of the poem? Why, if children and 'the very old' (line 8) 'enter' do 'most of us' just 'disappear'? Why do 'most of us' not just 'enter' like the others? What idea of death does this convey? For some, it conveyed a sense of lesser significance. The really significant deaths, it seemed, appear to be those of the 'harvesters' and 'islanders'. Only the islanders' Door of Water has 'beautiful names' on it. Those who work on the land and the sea seem to be given a special place, a special door. Or do the last two lines apply to all the doors and to all the deaths?:

> Beyond a lintel carved with beautiful names
> The sea yields to the bone, at last, its meaning.

The second half of the poem, like the first, takes the sting out of death. Like 'small wonderment' (line 3), 'tranquil sorrows' (line 9) suggests that there is peace in death, with a 'granary' (line 7) beyond – **what is this 'granary'?** Is this heaven? Or some other non-religious or pagan afterlife? What is a granary? – a granary is where grain is stored after being threshed – is it then an image of an afterlife? Or is this simply describing death in terms of natural cycles? Perhaps this is the clearest difference between the first and the second halves of the poem: the first half has no natural imagery and the second half compares death to the natural world, its rhythms and its 'meaning' (line 12). Gradually the poem identifies death with nature, almost literally, it seems, on a first and second reading. Finally, the poem suggests that there is 'meaning' in death if we can make this link with nature (and perhaps, implicitly, the link with religion?).

The idea, in this poem, that there are many kinds of death leaves the subject of death open to spiritual or emotional or more mundane interpretations. **Does this poem then imply that by seeing death in this way we can transform it from a fearful exit to a beautiful entrance?** Is this only possible for those who prepare to face death in this way? Is this poem then about ways people see death, or 'think of death'? Is this poem exploring the way our thoughts about death shape our experience of it? If so, this would mean that the 'Dove Door' could be the child's experience of its own death, because it knew nothing more; it had not developed a fear of death and would see only peace. This interpretation raises a further question for each reader: **Which of the deaths in this poem do we relate to most strongly?**

Can we prepare to have the death that suits us? Our group found that a final 'meaning' of the poem, the sense of death suiting the individual, could be something which made it easier to contemplate the deaths of those we love. In particular, the gentleness of 'yields' (line 12) and the relief in 'at last' (line 12) end the poem on the same note as 'small wonderment' (line 3) and 'tranquil sorrows' (line 9), although these last two seemed inappropriately gentle on a first reading. Finally, the harmony, the sense of things having an order, even in death, even if delicately balanced, was, for us, ultimately reassuring, moving and beautiful. This poem provided, for some, a glimpse of peace in death, and even of peace in thinking about it.

The gentleness of this poem, which began with 'Think of death, how it has many doors', contrasts dramatically with one of the best known poems about death, although, oddly, it also begins with an instruction:

> Do not go gentle into that good night,
> Old age should burn and rave at close of day;
> Rage, rage against the dying of the light.

No 'tranquil sorrows' here. Dylan Thomas's poem appears in the anthology *All in the End is Harvest*, which provides an introduction to each text, spelling out how each approaches the subject of death. Since this collection is subtitled *An Anthology for Those Who Grieve*, there was some concern in our group that Thomas's poem would be read by people who identified with the title but would find neither the relief nor comfort they might have been seeking in the poem. For example, any readers who knew they were going to die, or who knew someone close to them who was dying, would, it was suggested by some in our group, be disturbed by this view of death and dying. There was too much anger, it was felt, and this could be too unsettling for those still coming to terms with death. This could be an interesting talking point for other groups: **Is it appropriate to include/exclude rage or anger from discussions of death?** If this seems too general a question, perhaps placing it in a context would be helpful. There is also the related question of giving poems to patients to read: would either or both of these poems work well in that way?

The purpose of including this view of death and dying in the anthology is revealed in a brief introduction to the poem:

As well as recalling, and trying to find reconciliation with, the memory of those who rebelled against dying, this poem's power can surely also be harnessed in our anger **about** the death. Why should someone be allowed to disappear gently, quietly, without a feeling of outrage? And yet even the poet acknowledges death as 'that good night'. You may not at first face it gently, but maybe you do not have to fight it for ever.

> Whitaker, A. (ed.) (1992) *All in the End is Harvest: An Anthology for Those Who Grieve*, Longman & Todd, London, p. 30

According to this reading, although this poem starts in a very different tone, some of its ideas run parallel to points raised in our discussion of George Mackay Brown's poem. There is also an explicit echo of 'Most of us ... **Disappear**' in 'Why should someone be allowed to **disappear** gently'. While these two poems contrast so starkly in their opening lines and in tone, therefore, there are parallels in the movement from anger or bewilderment to peace and meaning.

Many other parallels are brought out in the general introduction to this anthology. Themes that emerge from writings on this subject, death, are defined here. This book could be a helpful resource both for groups working through texts on this subject and for facilitators looking for ideas and questions for discussion. The extensive range of readings and themes is likely to broaden the range of issues raised in any one group. For example, the book's introduction highlights recurring themes:

Yet there are common themes, ideas of potent imagery and meaning, which emerge again and again throughout this book. One is the theme of hope, hope that, however bad grief may be, it has a meaning; hope that all the good that can come out of love is not lost; hope that the meaning of life extends beyond life.

Another theme is the idea that, however dimly we comprehend it, everything relates to everything else; all is not chaos. Light and shade, pain and pleasure, love and loss are elements of a pattern whose details we perceive, even though we can never hope to perceive the whole....

And there is another theme which cuts across and includes the others, the theme of transcendence. This is, perhaps, the hardest to contain with words; it struggles and bolts to leap free. It develops out of despair into resignation, from resignation to surrender, from surrender to renunciation, from renunciation to acceptance and from acceptance to transcendence. In this process fear is transmuted into anger and anger into peace.   p. xi

Any of these 'common themes' could be the focus for discussion: **Have we seen these themes in the texts we have read?** Do we recognize these elements? Have we come across this progression from despair to peace in our reading? Are the terms of this progression different? interrupted? irrational? in some texts and contexts?

These two texts, George Mackay Brown's poem and Dylan Thomas's poem from the anthology, have emphasized the progression from anger to peace and in doing so have passed quickly over the despair which some would say is part of that progression and which others would argue is its most intense stage, depression and mental illness. These responses are dealt with in Janice Galloway's novel *The Trick is to Keep Breathing*, the story of a woman having a breakdown after the accidental death of her lover.

A longer extract from this novel than is printed here (pp. 18–23) was used to stimulate discussion and reflection in an undergraduate class on health promotion. A 2-hour session on medical humanities was used to give the students an opportunity to consider literature as a means of understanding the patient as a whole. What follows here is a summary of this session in outline form, along with comments and writings by participants in this discussion. The extract I selected shows an interaction between the woman who is experiencing a breakdown and the health visitor:

Extract from Janice Galloway's *The Trick is to Keep Breathing*

I get flustered at these times, but I know I'll manage if I try harder. These visits are good for me. Dr Stead sends this woman out of love. He insisted.

I said, I'm no use with strangers.

He said, But this is different. Health Visitors are trained to cope with that. He said she would know what to do; she would find me out and make me talk. **Make me** talk.

HAH

I'm putting on the kettle, still catching my breath when she comes in without knocking and frightens me. What if I had been saying things about her out loud? I tell her to sit in the living room so I can have time to think.

Tray

jug

sweeteners

plates

cups and saucers

another spoon

christ

the biscuits
the biscuits
the biscuits
I burst the wrap soundlessly and make a tasteful arrangement. I polish her tea-spoon on my cardigan band. No teapot. I make it in the cup, using the same bag twice, and take it through as though I've really made it in a pot and just poured it out. Some people are sniffy about tea-bags. It sloshes when I reach to push my hair back from falling in my eyes and I suddenly notice I am still wearing my slippers dammit.
Never mind. She smiles and says
Well!
This is to make out the tea is a surprise though it isn't. She does it every time. ... The chairs cough dust from under their sheets as she crosses her legs, think-ing her way into the part. By the time she's ready to start I'm grinding my teeth back into the gum.
Health Visitor: So, how are you/how's life/what's been happening/anything interesting to tell me/what's new?
Patient: Oh, fine/nothing to speak of.
I stir the tea repeatedly. She picks a piece of fluff off her skirt.
Health Visitor: Work. How are things at work? Coping?
Patient: Fine. [Pause] I have trouble getting in on time, but getting better.
I throw her a little difficulty every so often so she feels I'm telling her the truth.
I figure this will get rid of her quicker.   pp. 20–21

This session started with an introduction to medical humanities – aims, activities and the Glasgow group – followed by time for reading the extract. The main part of the session lasted one hour and followed the structure developed throughout this book:

Structure

Initial reflection: 5 minutes' private writing, in sentences, on the question: Do you think this health visitor is an effective facilita-tor? + pair-share, discussing writings and views (15 min)
Discussion: Group's responses to the question; other points raised by the text; focused discussion of text (30 min)
Further reflection: 5 minutes' writing, in sentences, on the ques-tion: What are the implications for health promotion?; Plenary and conclusions (15 min)
Total 60 min

Some readers may find this question too obvious – Do you think this health visitor is an effective facilitator?– of course, the health visitor appears to make some very basic mistakes. But the point of asking this question was to get the students to articulate their own definitions of effective facilitation and to justify their judgements by referring to the information they are given in the text. They might also, of course, have drawn on their own experience and learning. Whatever their frame of reference, and even within a class group, participants will define both 'effective' and 'facilitator' differently. In reading, they will make different interpretations of details in the text. This is the point of the apparently obvious question and it should be noted that there were both 'yes' and 'no' answers in this group – as there would probably be in other groups – and that both positions were well argued with reference to the text and to personal and professional experience.

An example of the 5 minutes' private writing on the question shows one participant taking the question at face value, while perhaps also opening up some of the areas for debate. Some of the references in this writing refer to the longer section we used in that discussion (pp. 18–23):

Question

Do you think this health visitor is an effective facilitator?

Five minutes' writing

I think the health visitor isn't an effective facilitator, based on details like not taking her coat off, trying to use examples of other people's misfortunes to enable talk, and giggling when she dribbles her tea, which seems oddly inappropriate. Talking too much. Too many routine questions. Not waiting for an answer. Yet this is not the 'worst' session, according to the thoughts of the 'patient'. The first was the worst and this therefore implies that some progress has been made, even if very little, through contact with the health visitor. So, maybe she is being effective, but only partially, and perhaps this is a realistic pace. Then there is the problem of point of view. This is the patient's point of view and that's subjective. So, she doesn't see the point of the visits and does, at the same time – i.e. she **knows** there's a point, logically, but also **knows**, i.e. thinks in her own terms, that this is not the way she will recover. So, it's a limited point of view. The health professional has to decide how best to change this point of view.

This writing reveals the participant's implicit definition of 'effectiveness' in this context. It also shows the complexity of the question, particularly when point of view is brought into the judgement. The writer has also engaged with the point of view of the patient, which was the primary goal of this session.

Writings were discussed, as usual, in a pair-share, with participants revealing as much or as little as they chose. This pairs work allowed participants safely to test out a few of their ideas before bringing them to the plenary.

The plenary began with one student recounting that she had had a friend who wouldn't speak, like the character in the novel, until one day she stopped speaking to her friend and her friend started speaking to her. Although this may seem to take a discussion of the extract off at a tangent, this was obviously an important parallel for this student, and an important lesson, concisely put, for the other students and lecturers to consider. The discussion continued, with both answers to the question – 'yes' and 'no' – presented by the students. Their answers were supported – after prompting from the facilitator – with references to the text, where relevant, and to personal or professional experience, where appropriate. Here is an outline of their main points:

Do you think this health visitor is an effective facilitator? – student answers: 'No' and 'Yes'

'No'
She makes her more anxious.
She's not helping her at all.
She's not there for long enough.
Picking fluff off her coat – she should be more attentive to the patient.
The question-and-answer seems routine – the dashes suggest any option would do.
She needs to help the patient relax.
She asks too many questions at once – not reflecting back, etc.
Comes across as a script – in fact, it is written out like one.
She misses the cues, e.g. can't get up in the morning.
'Lucky girl' [health visitor calls the patient] seems totally inappropriate, even sarcastic.
She goes in without knocking.
She doesn't find out what the patient is interested in.

'Yes'
The health visitor has had the effect of making the patient prepare for her visit.

She uses irony because she knows it appeals to this patient.
The patient wants to get better, so the health visitor has had an effect.
The patient knows she's got a problem.
She also knows herself that she is not trying.
The patient wants her to be there: 'She goes on munching, knowing I don't want her to be here/that I do want her to be here but I can't talk to her' (p. 22).
The patient has admitted she has a problem: 'I can't stop getting frantic about the house being clean' (p. 18).
A personal connection – between these two people – is not a realistic goal at this stage.

Each student put forward their own answer at some stage in this discussion, but there was also interaction among the students, as they responded to or questioned each other's views and judgements of effective/ineffective facilitation.

Finally, further reflection on this extract and the issues it had raised was prompted by a final question: **What are the implications for health promotion?** After their 5 minutes' writing, students raised a variety of implications in a short open discussion:

It's difficult to strike a balance between being professional and establishing a personal connection with a patient. Where do you draw the line?
You have to be able to wear different hats with different patients.
Clinical language is needed, but not to put people off.
In some situations you can't know anything about a patient's emotional responses, but you have to treat them as if they have some, treat them like a real person.
You also have to be able to protect yourself.
You have to find a 'meeting point' for you and the patient.

After this session, and after the medical humanities facilitator had left the room, the students were asked to produce an evaluation of the session in a structured group interview. This evaluative instrument was designed and managed by the subject lecturer. Here are their comments.

Structured group interview of students: evaluation of medical humanities

---

What did you expect from this afternoon's talk?

To be more scientific 'lecture' (formal) style, as opposed to 'informal' style used. Expected it to look more at the medico-scientific issues as related to humanities, rather than the other way round. A structured lecture not really that relevant to our profession.

What did you gain from this afternoon's experience?

Better insight into complexities of professional–client interactions. Helping us to see things from the patient's/client's stance rather than just the profession's stance.
A different viewpoint for the situation and also the different expectations of each individual.

What aspects of the subject of medical humanities might you use in your own professional practice?

Sharing experiences with other health-care workers. Could encourage interprofessional communication – breaking down barriers.
Understanding patients' attitudes and emotions and altering your own behaviour to complement the patient's.

Do you feel the material could have been presented in a better manner, and if yes, how?

No. Clear and distinct. Well-suited to audience.
No. Clear, straight to the point, very informal and easily understood.

Since this evaluation was neither designed nor managed by the medical humanities facilitator, nor was I present during this discussion, these comments can be taken as a useful appraisal of the students' experience of the session. Clearly, even in a first, one-off session these students did engage in useful reflection, in spite of the fact that they had not expected this to be one of the outcomes. They had reflected on their own roles and their relationships to patients. They had discussed some difficult issues, like the personal–professional balance, which would continue to recur in their professional lives. Finally, they had experienced these positive outcomes while discussing a text that raised professional issues related to a health visitor, when this was not their own profession. This suggests that the medical subject, or professional context, does not need exactly to match the context of a group for a medical humanities discussion to provoke reflection on professional issues.

To conclude, the subject of this chapter, death, may not appear explicitly in this extract from Galloway's novel, but then it might not appear, in reality, in discussions between patients and health professionals; it might remain in the background of the patient–carer interaction but nevertheless be of paramount importance to the patient. It may have particular effects in any interaction. What this extract has shown is the impact of the aftershocks caused by a traumatic death. What the students' evaluations of this discussion show is that this medical humanities discussion had provided insights, for them, into the complex processes of working with patients and working with each other. Medical humanities had been, for them, on this occasion, a mechanism for prompting reflection on personal and professional issues.

Further reflection

If the initial reflection in this chapter was prompted by the question, Did you follow the poem's initial instruction to 'think of death'?, this final reflective writing could go all the way back to the writing produced at the start of the session, in order to look back at it now from the vantage point of extended discussion:

Looking at your initial writing, do you find that you have followed the poem's instruction to 'think of death' in your writing?

Alternatively, this reflective writing could pull together the individual's responses to each part of the discussion:

Has a theme emerged in your talking and writing about these texts?

Summary

The texts used in this discussion have all dealt with the same subject. Each text develops its own perspective: the first presents a peaceful pattern and meaning in death; the second presents aggressive confrontation as the appropriate, if panicky, response; the third presents the painful effect of one death as the unravelling of life and mind. Each of these stimulated reflection on death. All stimulated the group's admiration for the writers.

The comparison of these texts prevented us from seeing death and bereavement in any one way. So many views were presented in the texts and by the participants in our discussion and by the students in theirs. For example, it was possible to consider in discussion and writing, and accept in context, different responses to death and dying: the response of mental illness, in Galloway's writing, or the stages in grieving, in *All in the End is Harvest*, or of natural rhythms and religious faith, in George Mackay Brown's 'Door of Water'. However, in our discussion no one response dominated over the others.

Extending this discussion

There are possibilities for extending and widening this discussion of death. There are links between some of the issues raised in this chapter and Chapter 6. For example, comparisons will occur to some readers with Douglas Dunn's *Elegies* and Butler and Rosenblum's account of how, as a couple, they dealt with cancer.

In our group we also planned a follow-up discussion, at the request of participants, which attempted to address other specific issues, such as euthanasia. This involved finding a different selection of readings, based on this expressed interest:

- 'Euthanasia on the last frontier'. *Independent*, **3.4.95**, which looked at the variety of motives for euthanasia and the potential risk to minorities and the ageing, and included international views on the subject

- 'Should you write a living will?' *Independent*, **4.4.95**, which included an example of a living will, or 'advance directive', and details of how it could or should be managed
- 'Closing time', Thomas Laqueur's long review of Sherwin Nuland's book *How We Die*, which includes discussion of the processes by which we die and the relative roles of ethics and biology in decisions about how we die.

In our group we found the discussion of death in a medical humanities mode paradoxically stimulating and moving. We also acknowledged that there had previously been few occasions to talk in a sustained and positive way about death. We therefore found that we identified with the need to talk about death and dying which was emphasized at the end of one of our readings:

Most people hope to pass on in their sleep, but this is not the way the average person dies. For many, death does not come with dignity, and when, or how, we choose. It may certainly comfort some, and help our carers, if we can prepare living wills while we are still well enough to mind what happens to us. At the very least, it's time we talked about it.   Independent, **4.4.95**

Having discussed the proposition that we had lost the 'art' of dying, the possibility was offered here of recovering some of that 'art' and certainly some of the responsibility for managing our own deaths. For some of us, not all, this had been the only forum for discussing this topic in this way.

8 Taking a stand: *Jurassic Park*

Taking a topical issue ● *Individual views* ● *Structures of media responses*
● *Comparison of texts – literary and non-literary* ● *What to do with*
unresolved issues?

Texts

---

1. Participants' writing on genetic engineering
2. *Jurassic Park*, a novel by Michael Crichton
3. Newspaper articles on genetic engineering
4. 'Stobhill' (poem) by Edwin Morgan

This chapter describes a process for exploring a topical subject in writing and discussion: genetic engineering has been topical in the sense that it has been in the news, providing articles and broadcasts for our discussions, and topical also in the sense that it is complex, bringing social, moral and ethical questions to what appears to be a highly advanced science. The pace of the development of genetic engineering has, in fact, outstripped the pace of the development of ethical thinking about it, of public discussion of it and, it could be argued, of appropriate forms of control for it. There could, therefore, be some unresolved issues here.

This might be a difficult and even unsettling discussion: there will be those who are not sure what they think about the issues, and some will find that unsettling; and there will be those who base their responses to the issues on personal, perhaps religious, beliefs, and they may find it difficult to be part of an open debate on the 'rights' and 'wrongs' when they have already made up their minds. This mixture of responses may be difficult for all concerned. It may present a new challenge for the facilitator.

This topic can therefore be effective for moving the group on from the territory covered in previous chapters. The facilitator will perhaps play a stronger role in not only encouraging participants to address issues which are genuinely challenging but also enabling them to deal with moral ambiguities. There will be no easy resolution of the issues. The facilitator can use the familiar framework for discussion as a 'safety net'.

As a topic for discussion genetic engineering worked well in our group, perhaps because it exposed so many layers and levels of views; it is one of those issues that people can approach from a number of angles. Both personal and professional questions can be raised by examples of genetic engineering in practice, while literary treatments can focus on the human factor, which is often neglected in discussions about and, some would argue, in the development of genetic engineering.

The structure of this chapter is, like previous chapters, based on a framework for the process of group discussion: initial reflection, discussion, further reflection. The aim of following this structure over several chapters is to make it gradually more and more familiar to the reader who may be thinking either of starting a medical humanities group or of using some of this material in their teaching.

Variations on this structure are, of course, infinite and this framework is therefore to be taken as a guide. Other frameworks may, of course, develop in the work of a group; the idea here is to establish as familiar one framework while introducing a variety of texts, issues and questions. Different routes through the material are suggested here. Precise timings are therefore not given in this chapter, in order to allow for flexibility.

The inclusion of participants' writings in the list of 'texts' at the start of this chapter is intended to foreground them for this discussion; it could be that participants' views on the subject of genetic engineering will shape the discussion on this occasion.

A starting point is suggested for the initial reflection stage, in the form of general questions raised by participants in our discussion. The overall aim of this chapter, therefore, is to provide a flexible framework for other groups' discussions, since other groups may not choose to discuss the same issues as our group, but facilitators could structure the discussion in the same way as I did – if structure is needed, that is.

Initial reflection

What *is* genetic engineering?
What do I think about these examples of genetic engineering?

Most people in our group had read and/or heard about a number of specific cases of genetic engineering, cases which seemed to us to have involved different kinds of genetic manipulation and different motives:

- There was the case of a woman who wanted to have a child in her fifties, after she had had a career.
- There was the case of a black woman who wanted her child to be white, because she believed that it would have a better chance in life.
- There was the case of the isolation of the 'gay gene', which presents the opportunity to identify homosexuals, a prospect which was quickly followed by predictions that everyone would soon be carrying 'genetic passports'.

These examples – i.e. details of these cases – appeared to us to have received more attention in the media than any debates for or against the advancement of this science. The cases presented strange new possibilities which had, as far as we knew, never been feasible before and for this reason, of course, they made good news.

We read a number of newspaper articles for additional information on the science behind these applications. Some newspapers did begin to raise questions about the ethics of these cases. However, although we did not find any arguments in favour of developing this science at any cost, without knowing the consequences, this did come up in other readings and in our discussions.

At the start of our discussion some participants admitted that these issues were so complex that they did not know where they stood:

> I don't know what I think about these things ....
> I really haven't made up my mind.
> I'm not sure ... what do I think about this?

Some held the belief that any form of genetic engineering was wrong, because it was 'like playing God'. Some believed that is was wrong because, like abortion, it offered the possibility of terminating what they saw as life in its earliest form. Others felt that arguments for or against genetic engineering would hinge, for them, on the definition of when life could be said to begin. So, even although some participants had still to make up their minds about genetic engineering, deeply held beliefs were brought into play immediately.

Initial writing gave participants a means to express these beliefs. It also provided time to react to the issues, to begin to address any of the many questions raised here or to explore responses to a particular case. The tentative nature of these initial comments were, it is perhaps worth pointing out for other groups and potential participants, a form of acknowledgement of the difficulty of decision making in this area.

An alternative writing activity could be to summarize one or more of the readings. This writing – again for 5 minutes – could be either private or for sharing, depending on the nature and/or wishes of the group. Participants could decide for themselves here. In any case, the writing could provide material for discussion.

Familiarity with this type of writing activity will probably have made it less intimidating to those participants who have been meeting for some time. However, while it has become familiar, it may serve a different function here; private writing may create a 'space' for participants to express their own tentative views on this particularly challenging subject. The writing may become the space where they can express views freely and separately from others, without being swamped by others' views.

Discussion

This section roughly follows the structure of our discussion and includes its key elements, in order to help others who may choose this topic for discussion:

- notes on each text;
- questions that came up in our discussion;
- summaries of arguments developed by participants in our group.

In order to encourage exploration of this topic from a number of different angles I selected three different kinds of text as readings:

- **faction** – a mixture of fact and fiction – which presented some background information and a dramatization of some of the issues;
- **newspaper articles on genetic engineering**, which provided more factual information and summarized a wide range of views, yet presented each case as if it raised discrete issues, distinct from other cases;
- **a poem** on a hospital incident in which an aborted fetus, discarded as waste, was found to be alive just before it was to be put in the incinerator.

The 'faction' text was *Jurassic Park*, a story where genetic engineering is used to recreate prehistoric species using DNA recovered from blood from a mosquito preserved in amber. This novel raises a wide range of issues: commercialization, the ethics of scientific advancement and practical and ethical controls. Many of the recurring issues in genetic engineering are summarized in the novel's introduction:

First extract from Michael Crichton's *Jurassic Park* – Introduction: 'The InGen Incident'

The late twentieth century has witnessed a scientific gold rush of astonishing proportions: the headlong and furious haste to commercialize genetic engineering. This enterprise has proceeded so rapidly – with so little outside commentary – that its dimensions and implications are hardly understood at all.
Biotechnology promises the greatest revolution in human history. By the end of this decade, it will have outdistanced atomic power and computers in its effect on our everyday lives. In the words of one observer, 'Biotechnology is going to transform every aspect of human life: our medical care, our food, our health, our entertainment, our very bodies. Nothing will ever be the same again. It's literally going to change the face of the planet'. p. ix

The fascination of genetic engineering – for experts and non-experts alike – is effectively captured in this novel. The associated sensationalism may create an illusion of public involvement in the debate. The dominant forces of commercialism, however, along with limited public involvement, expose the real motives behind this particular example of genetic engineering. The underdevelopment of an ethical framework, finally, is pinpointed here in general terms and later in more specific terms by one of the characters, a chaos mathematician.

This introduction to the novel is written in a factual way, as if making factual statements about genetic engineering and in a reporting style: 'First ... Second ... Third'. For our group, because these issues did appear in the press at the time of our discussion this summary seemed, in fact, to ring true. It lays out a number of the core issues and constructs a critical, yet at the same time seductive, view of genetic engineering by depicting both its risks and its fantastic potential. We recognized that the language of sensationalism heightened the tone of this description and, potentially, of the debate: 'It's literally going to change the face of the planet'. This raised a question later in our discussion – which other groups may raise at this stage – of whether or not this is simply sensationalization or whether genetic engineering does, in fact, have the potential to 'change the face of the planet'. And if it does have this potential what are the implications ... for us ... now?

This balance between fact and speculation make up the faction that is Michael Crichton's forte. (For his 'faction' treatment of a medical subject see his early novel *A Case of Need*.) This form of writing is perhaps entirely appropriate to genetic engineering, where so much has been achieved in scientific terms but so little has been worked out in human terms, and where some of the specific cases **do** seem fantastic.

The chaos mathematician, mentioned above, raises questions about the implications of genetic engineering, raising, in the process, broader questions about scientific methods and scientists' values. In fact, his mathematical equations show that the Jurassic Park 'experiment' is bound to fail. In conversation with another scientist, a palaeontologist (in the second extract used in our discussion), he expounds his views:

Second extract from Michael Crichton's *Jurassic Park*

'Scientists are actually preoccupied with accomplishment. So they are focused on whether they can do something. They never stop to ask if they **should** do something. They conveniently define such considerations as pointless. If they don't do it, someone else will. Discovery, they believe, is inevitable. So they just try to do it first. That's the game in science. Even pure scientific discovery is an aggressive, penetrative act. It takes big equipment, and it literally changes the world afterward. Particle accelerators scar the land, and leave radioactive byproducts. Astronauts leave trash on the moon. There is always some proof that scientists were there, making their discoveries. Discovery is always a rape of the natural world. Always.

'The scientists want it that way. They have to stick their instruments in. They have to leave their mark. They can't just watch. They can't just appreciate. They can't just fit into the natural order. They have to make something unnatural happen. That is the scientist's job, and now we have whole societies that try to be scientific.' ...

Ellie said, 'Don't you think you're overstating – '

'What does one of your excavations look like a year later?'

'Pretty bad,' she admitted.

'You don't replant, you don't restore the land after you dig?'

'No.'

'Why not?'

She shrugged. 'There's no money, I guess....'

'There's only enough money to dig, but not to repair?'

'Well, we're just working in the badlands....'

'Just the badlands', Malcolm said, shaking his head. 'Just trash. Just byproducts. Just side effects ... I'm trying to tell you that scientists **want** it this way. They want byproducts and trash and scars and side effects. It's a way of reassuring themselves. It's built into the fabric of science, and it's increasingly a disaster.'

'Then what's the answer?'

'Get rid of the thintelligent ones. Take them out of power.'

'But then we'd lose all the advances – '

'What advances?' Malcolm said irritably. 'The number of hours women devote to housework has not changed since 1930, despite all the advances. All the vacuum cleaners, washer-dryers, trash compactors, garbage disposals, wash-and-wear fabrics ... Why does it still take as long to clean the house as it did in 1930?' ...

'Because there haven't been any advances', Malcolm said. 'Not really. Thirty thousand years ago, when men were doing cave paintings at Lascaux, they worked twenty hours a week to provide themselves with food and shelter and clothing. The rest of the time, they could play, or sleep, or do whatever they wanted. And they lived in a natural world, with clean air, clean water, beautiful trees and sunsets. Think about it. Twenty hours a week. Thirty thousand years ago.'

Ellie said, 'You want to turn back the clock?'
'No,' Malcolm said. 'I want people to wake up. We've had four hundred years of modern science, and we ought to know by now what it's good for, and what it's not good for. It's time for a change.'
'Before we destroy the planet?' she said.
He sighed, and closed his eyes. 'Oh dear,' he said. 'That's the **last** thing I would worry about.'   pp. 284–285

The contrast between startling discoveries and far from startling human motives is one of the key movements in this story. That the mathematician has worked out that this experiment is bound to fail is beautifully ironic.

Chaos theory is a bit beyond me.

His calculations use chaos maths, which is explained progressively in the course of this novel, each chapter opening with a diagram. A series of fractals illustrates Malcolm's calculations. This sequence of images represents the step-by-step disintegration of the Jurassic Park plan, the gradual build-up of errors, short-cuts, corruption and unforeseen events, culminating in what becomes an increasingly predictable disaster.

However, what taxed us even more than chaos maths was the logic used by the scientists involved in this project to support their assumption that their genetically engineered new creatures and the reinvented environments could all be precisely controlled, like some laboratory experiment. In our group we acknowledged that these scientists were to be credited, like their non-fictional counterparts, with an imaginative leap of faith, persistence, creativity and invention in their research, but this narrative also exposed, for us, the lack of care and control that can come with commercialization.

Ethical issues, then, are raised by this character, Malcolm the mathematician. He explicitly raises the 'is *versus* ought' question: **Just because something is possible does this mean that we ought to do it?** His monologue is less a critique of commercialization – which was the aim of the novel's introduction – and more a moral commentary on scientific processes as he sees them. What he questions is the unquestioning drive towards an illusion, as he sees it, of scientific progress, whatever the cost. The implications of scientific advances are, he argues, rarely, if ever, part of the scientific design. It is precisely this lack of reflection on the implications of scientific developments that leads him to raise other questions about controls.

This character provides ample material, in this extract and at other points in the novel, for further discussion among groups, either among scientists or among non-scientists. Along with the explicit questions about scientific thinking and working methods there are implicit questions about the education of scientists and perhaps also about the education of other specialist groups. As scientists and others become more and more specialized, it seems, they spend less and less time considering the implications of their work. Questions of how to achieve a particular goal overtake questions about whether the goal is good or bad. At what point does this kind of thinking develop in a professional career (if we agree that it does)? Is it only likely to happen to researchers? Or are specialists by definition thinking only of their specialism?

Is there a specialist-ethics gap?
And, if so, where does it start?

- in Michael Crichton's view?
- in the character Malcolm's view?
- in your own view?

How do we bridge the specialist-ethics gap?

The root of the problem, for the character Malcolm, very clearly lies in what he calls 'thintelligence':

He's an engineer.... They're both technicians. They don't have intelligence. They have what I call 'thintelligence'. They see the immediate situation. They think narrowly and they call it 'being focused'. They don't see the surround. They don't see the consequences. That's how you get an island like this. From thintelligent thinking. Because you cannot make an animal and not expect it to act **alive**. To be unpredictable. To escape. But they don't see that.   p. 284

The problem, in his view, is a kind of structural separation of science and its context: in the rush to advance, scientists have either simply lost the ability to see the context of their work or do not have the ability to do so. A third interpretation could be that the context is considered but is disregarded in the race to be first; it is simply not as important as being first. Where 'being first' is paramount, side-effects can more easily be ignored and/or explained away, in terms of some 'greater good'.

This extract from the novel brings a new meaning to the word 'singleminded': Malcolm has argued that scientists are literally single-minded, in the sense that they are driven by a single goal, focused, words which, in another context, would seem quite positive but which he uses here to characterize what he sees as a weakness in thinking. This reversal of meanings, along with Malcolm's other opinionated, perhaps overstated, propositions, may strike a cord with readers or, alternatively, may hit a nerve. The fact that much of what he says does in fact turn out to be accurate may simply add fuel to the debate about his views:

Has Malcolm overstated the case against science and scientists?
What is the basis for your answer?
Do you agree or disagree with him because of

- events in the novel?
- your own knowledge and/or experience?

Whether we agree or disagree with Malcolm he has raised a number of ethical questions:

Should we, as a species, or they, as scientists, do this science?
What are the pros and cons of genetic engineering?
If we have not fully considered these then how can we decide?
Are scientists trained not to ask these questions?

In our discussions, scientists were becoming typecast, as in Malcolm's critique of them, and we began to explore our own and each other's beliefs and prejudices about scientists. There was a position taken by some in our group that faulted scientists in general – or in genetic engineering in particular – for seeing these as lower-order questions, as less important than the science itself: what matters in scientific research is results. We recognized that these ethical questions are not the questions that are regularly taken into the lab for scrutiny and discussion. We acknowledged that there may be no educational or professional forum in which scientists can consider their own answers to such questions. We argued about perceived value judgements, based on perceptions of a hierarchy which allows some scientists to see themselves as most qualified to make or to ignore ethical decisions even if in practice they have had very little experience of reflecting on ethical issues. And, being fair, we considered that this last point may be true of other professional groups.

Educators in our group took up the related issue of discipline-based training. There was a view that this is where boundaries between subjects and hierarchies among and within professions are created. The training of an elite group for the top of the hierarchy, the group which allegedly need not question its motives and does not allow anyone else to do so, was seen as having obvious risks.

We also discussed Malcolm's view that scientists are motivated by a desire to leave their mark whatever the cost. There were plenty of examples of this competitive urge and a general awareness in our group that having the competitive edge is, in some areas of research, worth billions. We also knew of cases where side-effects had been presented as the lesser of two evils, in the interests of marketing a new product. We also discussed the apparently widespread belief – or illusion? – that new discoveries always represent 'progress'.

This text, therefore, generated many important ethical questions, questions about the rights and wrongs of science, about motives in pursuing scientific research and about reasons for valuing scientific 'results':

What is science good for and what makes 'good science?'
Who should decide the answer to these questions?
How can we make any kind of change and who listens to us?
Is there such a thing as 'wrong' values?

These questions appeared to be of equal interest to those who were engaged in science and to those who were not. Those in the group who were being encouraged by their professional bodies and employing institutions to initiate research, perhaps for the first time, appreciated the opportunity to air their views on this drive to research at all costs. First-time researchers in the group could wrestle with some of the questions which this new demand had raised for them. Interestingly, there are some parallels between their questions and Malcolm's:

First-time researchers' questions

Why are we being asked/pressurized to do research?
Should we be doing this at all?
How will we find the time?
Why do we have to do it in our spare time?
What support will I get?

Malcolm's particular concern is to profess the importance of context, but Ellie appears never to have given it a second thought, affirming that her research funding does not include consideration of its human or social implications or side-effects. At this point our discussion cycled back to the impact of the education process, rather than of the funding bodies, in shaping people's thinking, their values and their professional practice. A number of people held the view that there was a systematic exclusion of the humanities from scientific education. In fact, it was this exclusion which, they felt, created the need for medical humanities; it could be used to create dialogue between the sciences and the humanities.

The sciences and the humanities may be brought together by a facilitator who is willing and able to cross disciplines, to build a bridge between the disciplines and not necessarily simply to exercise literary expertise. Perhaps this means that the medical humanities facilitator need not necessarily be someone who sees herself or himself primarily as an expert at all, but someone who is not 'singleminded', someone who is prepared to create links between the disciplines and between the people who work in them.

The facilitator, therefore, should be someone who knows their way around a literary text, so to speak, but who is not exclusively literary in their approach to texts. If this person is able to stray into other territory then so much the better; this will give him/her an understanding of other professions. An ability not to be territorial is a key skill here; the ability to enable others not to be territorial about their disciplines or professions is also valuable. Since the participants' starting point may well be, understandably, territoriality, perhaps this very point should be a 'required' talking point for the group.

Links between academic disciplines are difficult enough to create even for the purposes of interdisciplinary study. The disciplines are systematically separated into different courses and separate departments. The infrastructure of devolved budgets may further inhibit interaction. Yet interaction between the disciplines can take place quite easily – and cheaply – through the interaction of texts from different disciplines. Bringing together the various 'voices' of scientific and literary texts is one way of creating this interaction.

Taking a topical issue is one way of latching on to the interests of both scientists and others, since scientific and non-scientific information will be made available in easily accessible forms through the media. Genetic engineering, the mapping of human genes and the identification of particular genes, was chosen as an example of a topical issue for discussion because it is a powerful topic which is likely to continue to appear in the media. The implications and potential applications will continue to raise critical questions about the delicate balance between individual freedom of choice and social codes and controls.

This broader range of issues was explicitly raised, if only as an afterthought, in several short articles we read, including leader articles, from a selection of newspapers. Our purpose in reading these articles was to find further information about genetic engineering. But we also analysed them as texts, not just as 'facts' but as interpretations of the subject, not quite in the same way as literary texts but with their own level of subjectivity and vested interests.

In these writings a pattern emerged; genetic engineering was a story of scientific advance first and reflection on implications second. A number of articles reported events in precisely this way, and in some cases individual researchers themselves announced in these articles that ethical issues could be explored after the discovery had been made, as if the discovery were a trigger for ethical discussion. Examples of this structure have been highlighted in the following extracts from articles we read. Notes for discussion are also provided here:

Extracts from newspaper articles on genetic engineering and related issues

Advances in the mapping of human genes will mean that within 50 years people could be given a 'genetic passport' telling them what diseases they are likely to suffer from, a professor of molecular biology predicted today.
Ethical and legal debate needed to begin now on who would be given such information and whether insurance companies or employers should be allowed to discriminate against people on the basis of their future health.

Guardian, **2.9.93**

The discovery of a 'gene for homosexuality' **will open a Pandora's Box in terms of the ethical and legal implications**....
Dr Hamer emphasizes that one gene, or a group of genes, is not designed to test for sexual orientation....
Nevertheless, he is concerned that this and other work to unravel the entire genetic makeup of humans ... will raise **important ethical questions that have yet to be addressed**.

Independent, **16.7.93**

Because homosexual uncles and male cousins of the gay subjects were raised in different households, the scientists hypothesized a genetic factor on the X chromosome was responsible....
'Once we have the gene, we'll be able to understand it', he said.

Independent, **16.7.93**

The point about making the discovery first and then considering implications – 'Once we have the gene, we'll be able to understand it' – appears logical, but is it impossible to reflect on implications before discovery? The social context for these research questions appears to have been ignored, although the social context would appear to raise some very serious questions in this example.

Questions we had raised and discussed up to this point were quite general, but examples of genetic engineering raised, for us, questions specific to each case:

Genetic engineering: specific questions

What is the social context for developing a technique to determine a person's sexuality?
How will society benefit from this discovery?
How will individuals benefit from this discovery?
Why is so much time, effort and research money being allocated to this subject?
Surely homosexuals have already developed the ability to identify themselves as homosexuals, or not, as they wish?
Why do we need a technique for someone else to identify them?
Does the search for a gay gene rest on the presupposition that only a select few are 'carriers' of the gay gene?
Have the researchers considered the possibility that there are gay genes in many people, or perhaps in most people, or in everyone, and that only social and legal sanctions have made people suppress their genes?

We also considered the potential value – to society and to the individual – of isolating other genes: why not isolate the gene for murderers?; why not isolate the gene for artists? Knowing the gene for artists would allow us to sponsor one or two in their work at an early stage. What about isolating the gene for great humanitarians – defined by their actions? – then we could make sure that there were more of them around. Or would we? We might then be able to combine these findings with research on the gay gene to find out how many gays and lesbians had been great humanitarians. All of these suggestions rely on one huge assumption: that we would be able to control not only the genes we had isolated but also the uses of this technology: **Should we assume that we will be able to programme genes in this way? Is this development desirable?**

Some participants felt that the answers to these questions were quite obvious: there is obviously a hidden agenda, in genetic engineering in general and in isolating the gene for homosexuality in particular. That this is a social agenda was seen by some as deeply ironic, given that this would, presumably, be hotly denied by the scientists, who would, presumably, maintain that this is 'pure' research. Others added that, while the answers to some of these questions might be obvious, the questions were not being asked often enough, if at all: there was a need to open up the discussion on social engineering which might, by design or by default, be the outcome of this application of genetic engineering.

'Certain applications are obvious,' was also the view of one researcher who could foresee the development of a 'test for homosexuality' as one potential development of his research that he would strenuously resist:

Once the gene is found it would be possible to develop a test that could help detect carriers of the genetic trait. But Dr Hamer warned that if such a test were devised, it would be no more than 50 per[cent] accurate in identifying homosexuality; little better than relying on a toss of a coin....

Dr Hamer said he would oppose the development of a blood test [for homosexuality] at every opportunity and would try to block companies that attempted to invent a test based on his work.... **'Certain applications are obvious'.** *Independent,* **23.2.94**

The statement that 'Certain applications are obvious' raises the obvious question of why they have not been thought through in advance, if they are so obvious. Again the applications and implications appear to have taken second place. The difference here is that the scientist has revealed that it is possible to anticipate applications, implying that it is possible simply to ignore them while progressing with scientific work. In our discussion we puzzled over the prospect of scientists who are not, after all, 'disabled' by their 'singleminded' education but who are deliberately ignoring the implications of their work. Some participants felt that this was irresponsible, a moral 'sin of omission'.

The potential for misuse of genetic research, of which the researcher quoted in the previous extract was acutely aware, was present at every stage in our discussion.

In the days and weeks after this discussion, we noticed that other scientific developments were reported in a similar pattern: Innovations first ... and implications second.

Some articles consisted of an announcement of completed research and/or of new products, followed by what appeared to be an invitation to us all to consider its implications:

Psychiatrists are urging family doctors to resist pressure from patients wanting the anti-depressant Prozac....

More than nine million people worldwide have taken the drug, about half of them in the United States, where it is being absorbed into the national culture....

'The observation of Prozac's effects may well be genuine; **it is the interpretation which needs to be looked at.'** *Independent on Sunday,* 31.10.93

Similarly, a report on investigations of radiation discharges and their impact on the environment revealed that some saw this as a legitimate method of inquiry; the research was paramount, whatever the side-effects:

'One of the principal and, I believe, most effective methods of carrying out these investigations, is indeed to **use radioactivity and discharge it and find out what happens to it.**
'This leads to information a great deal more sound than that which can be obtained by small-scale and laboratory experiments.' [John Dunster, Board member of the International Commission on Radiological Protection]
Mr Mike Townsley, of Scottish anti-nuclear group Scram, said ... 'The implications are horrendous and display a complete disregard for public safety'.

The Herald, **23.7.93**

Anyone living in the vicinity of the radioactive installation in question would presumably see this as taking the 'do-it-first-think-about-it-later' method more than a little too far. Even those of us who do not live within 'discharging distance' of an installation found this an unbelievably dangerous strategy.

As a final example of this 'innovations first, implications second' pattern of thinking, working or writing, without looking too far, we came across cases where medical advances had literally been put into practice without any consideration of the ethical, legal and social implications:

Fast action by a New York surgeon who removed sperm from the corpse of a man 13 hours after he died **may lead to the procedure becoming commonplace in the United States, in spite of unanswered ethical questions....**
The procedure raises the question of conferring paternity on a man after his death and without consent.   *Independent*, **26.1.95**

The words 'fast action' suggest a brave, adventurous and well-intentioned response to a crisis situation, validating the surgeon's spontaneous medical advance. The leap from the one-off crisis to the 'commonplace' is made within one sentence. The mixture of speculation about the innovation and concerns about the implications in this extract is very familiar; it has been a feature of many other extracts quoted in this chapter.

This text almost exactly mirrors a paragraph from *Jurassic Park*, a paragraph which seemed, to some, fantastic on a first reading:

The late twentieth century has witnessed a scientific gold rush of astonishing proportions: the headlong and furious haste to commercialize genetic engineering. This enterprise has proceeded so rapidly – with so little outside commentary – **that its dimensions and implications are hardly understood at all....**
Scientists are actually preoccupied with accomplishment. So they are focused on whether they can do something. They never stop to ask if they **should** do something.   pp. ix and 284

Both paragraphs have the same three components:

• speed, in 'fast action' and 'gold rush ... furious haste';

- innovations becoming 'commonplace' and 'commercialize[d]';
- ethical questions which have been ignored.

Comparing two paragraphs: *Jurassic Park* **and the** *Independent* article

What are the implications of these similarities?
Are they simply coincidental?
Is the faction of *Jurassic Park* moving closer to the truth?
Or does genetic engineering invite this kind of speculation in style of writing and in surgical practice?

Perhaps the similarity in style is due to the process of speculating, thinking ahead to the potential of new techniques in genetic engineering, thinking about what they **could** do, and delaying, as a fictional character would have reminded us, in thinking about whether or not we **should** do so.

Questions for discussion here could also arise from issues identified in the media, or the pattern identified in this reporting or the issues selected for discussion. Participants might, again, appreciate some time to reflect on this collection of articles (since the group will have read each of the articles in full, not just the short extracts reproduced in this chapter).

Participants and facilitators can provide their own selection of articles, summaries of broadcasts and conversations and examples from their own experiences. It might be helpful at this stage to suggest that participants highlight what for them is the main issue in genetic engineering:

What, for you, is the main issue here?
If you cannot isolate one issue, what are your main concerns?

In our discussion we tended not to isolate one case of genetic engineering from another; the discussion tended to move from one case to another. Common issues therefore emerged across all these examples:

Issues emerging in discussion

Motives
Controls
Contextualization
Commercialization.

Some in our group felt that all of these issues should be included in scientific education. Others questioned the role of research councils and companies: should they have a stronger steer on the ethics of research, or should another, independent body oversee their practice?

Our conclusion, perhaps not emerging coherently from our discussion, was that values must still be attached to humanity. We established as our common ground, whatever our views on individual cases, that humanity should be the basis of moral codes for research, as for anything else. These generalizations may seem to be clutching at straws; our conclusions remained undefined in this way. Our aim was to recover some core of moral values that we held in common. In our own way we felt that we had achieved this, without negotiating a precise definition of such terms as 'humanity'. This was reassuring, since it would be disturbing – or perhaps absurd? – to expect that the complexity of genetic engineering could remove all our moral constants.

While we realized this conclusion would not be adequate for an Ethics Committee – not that all of their conclusions were adequate for us – we felt that there was value in establishing common values because they had helped us to return to simple principles. (We remained very clear that we did not agree on some principles.) So, the final stage of this discussion was a statement of common values, with the emphasis on 'common' rather than precise definition of 'values'.

We remained unsure of the extent to which this principle, putting 'humanity' first, could be implemented in genetic engineering. Certain questions remained unanswered:

Is humanity put first in genetic engineering?
Is it possible to establish principles and appraise individual cases?
Isn't this meant to be happening already?

With these questions still in the air, we moved on to our final text, a poem chosen for discussion alongside *Jurassic Park* and the articles on genetic engineering because it deals with abortion. This turned out to have been a fortuitous choice, since it only emerged in our discussion that abortion occupied, for some participants, the same territory as genetic engineering, that is, they saw it as morally wrong for the same reasons.

This poem describes an incident in a Glasgow hospital: an aborted fetus was found to be alive just before being put in the incinerator. The poem brings together the points of view of the doctor, the boilerman, the mother, the father and the porter. Each person gives his/her version of the story and his/her sense of its rights and wrongs. They do this in what appears to be a monologue, as if defending their own actions. Each point of view is represented in the individual style of the speaker. Each has 30 lines or so and extracts of about a dozen lines from each are included here.

Many of the issues we had been discussing in this session were brought together here. Many of the different points of view are also voiced here, as different characters in the poem raise the issues which concern them most. Various social contexts are included.

Alternatively, could it be that the characters all share core values, but that this is obscured by their very different ways of expressing them?

Extract from Edwin Morgan's poem 'Stobhill'

The Doctor
Yes, I agreed to perform the abortion.
The girl was under unusual strain.
I formed the opinion that for personal reasons
and home circumstances her health would suffer
if pregnancy was not terminated....
These factors left me in no doubt.
Accordingly I delivered her seven months baby
without complications. It was limp and motionless.
I was satisfied there was no life in it.
Normal practice was followed: it was placed
in a paper disposal bag and sent
to the incinerator. Later to my surprise
I was told it was alive. It was then returned
and I massaged its chest and kept it warm.
It moved and breathed about eight hours.
Could it have lived? I hardly think so.
You call it a disturbing case? Disturbing
is a more emotive word than I would choose
but I take the point....

The Boilerman
Ay well, the porter brought this bag doon
(he'd come fae the operatin theatre like)
an he sayed it wis fur burnin....
...ah gote the fire up,
ah starts throwin bags in the incinerator,
an ah'm luftin this wee bag an
ah hear a sorta whimperin – cryin like –
an ah can feel somethin breathin
through the paper. Whit did ah dae?
Ah pit it on a binch, near the hote pipes.
An ah goes up thae sterrs fur the porter.
Asks him, What wis in that bag?
He says, A foetus. Ah says, What's that?

A kiddy, he says. D'ye ken it's alive? ah says.
He says, Yes. Ah says, It's a bluidy shame.
But the sleekit bugger never let dab
when he brought the bag. All he sayed wis burn it
and that's the God's truth. It's bad enough
whit the doctors dae, but he'd have been a murderer
if ah hadny heard the wean cryin...

The Mother

I've no idea who the father is.
I took a summer job in a hotel
in the Highlands, there was a party, I
got drunk, it must have happened then
but I remember nothing. When I knew
I was pregnant I was almost crazy,
it seemed the end of everything.
My father – it was impossible,
you have no idea what he is like,
he would certainly have turned me out
and made my mother's life unbearable
if it wasn't unbearable before....
I wanted to say that I – that my actions
are not very good and I don't defend them,
but I could not have the baby,
I just could not, you do see?
And now I never want to have one,
that's what it's done to me. I'm sick
of thinking, regretting, wishing, blaming.
I've gone so dead I see it all
like pulled from someone else's womb....

The Father

Did she? Did she? I'm not really surprised
I'm really not. Vodka, rum, gin –
some night yon was. Was it me?
Was it my bairn? Christ, I don't know,
it might have been, I had her all right –
but there was three of us you know –
at least three ...

The Porter

Ah know ah tellt them lies at the enquiry.
Ah sayed ah thought the wean wis dead
when ah took it tae the incinerator.
Ah didny think the wean wis dead,
but ah didny ken fur shair, did ah?
It's no fur me tae question the doctors....
... Everybody wants

tae come doon on me like a tonna bricks.
Ah canny go aboot openin disposal bags –
if ah did ah'd be a nervous wreck....
... Well ah'm no in court noo.
Don't answer nothin incriminatin, says the sheriff.
And that's good enough for yours truly.
And neither ah did, neither ah did,
neither ah did, neither ah did.   Edwin Morgan

ah = I; bairn = child; binch = bench; canny = cannot; dae = do; didny = didn't; doon = down; fae = from; fur shair = for sure; hadny = hadn't; hote = hot; ken = know; let dab = revealed what he knew; luftin = lifting; noo = now; pit = put; sheriff = judge of Scottish lower court; sleekit = sly; tellt = told; thae sterrs = those stairs; wean = child; wis = was; wis fur = was for; yon = that

The doctor's monologue is first. He gives a professional account of the case, referring to the child mainly as 'it', and seeks to detach emotion from the situation. There are no doubts or dilemmas here – 'These factors left me in no doubt'. A procedure has been performed and an unusual result has created an aberration for which the doctor, by his own account, cannot be held responsible. This last point seems, above all, what he is concerned to convey.

The initial 'yes' implies that the context is a dialogue and later the doctor refers to 'you' – 'You call it a disturbing case?' – and distances himself from the point of view of the person he is speaking to: 'Disturbing/ is a more emotive word than I would choose/ but I take the point.'

The combination of clinical details and this dispassionate response to someone else's emotional reaction shows that the doctor is very effective at managing his own emotional responses. The passive voice is as useful for disguising, as the active voice is useful for clarifying, exactly who did what:

Passive voice (in the poem)

> ... **it was placed**
> in a paper disposal bag and **sent**
> to the incinerator.

Active voice (an alternative)

> ... **I placed it**
> in a paper disposal bag and **sent it**
> to the incinerator.

His sensitivity to the predicament of the mother conveys some sympathy, although his revelation that the woman's father was a doctor has a hint of 'closing the ranks' motivation about it. This detail does, however, give the events some social context.

What is the tone of the doctor's speech? How would they sound if he said them aloud? Tone is often revealing of motives and concerns. Is the doctor being patronizing in a defensive way or in a superior way ... or not at all? What tone is he intending to strike? What tone do you hear?

- Tired but well-meaning?
- Arrogant?
- Patronizing?
- Sensitive?
- Helpful?
- Impatient?

Whatever our interpretation of his tone it is clear that the doctor not only sees this case as closed but also sees his own speech as answering any remaining questions.

The boilerman's account provides further details of what exactly happened to the fetus. From his point of view the event is shocking. Unlike the doctor, this man has no way of accounting for events, or of reasoning them out. The fact that he does not know the meaning of the word 'foetus' shows the gulf between his world and the doctor's, although if it was making the noises he described then presumably he had some idea of what was in the bag. One question raised by his account is **why did he not look inside the bag when he felt the child breathing and heard it whimpering?** Perhaps this is not the first time this has happened? Or was he so shocked that he could not do any-thing without talking to the porter? Or was he trying to cover himself by blaming someone else?

He reveals that he does know what the doctors do – 'It's bad enough/ whit the doctors dae'. He does not apparently see them as at fault in any way, either for 'what they do' in abortions or for this par-ticular incident. His anger is directed at the porter for letting the child get this far, when he knew it was still alive. Perhaps the boilerman rec-ognizes that he is more likely to be blamed than the doctor and is sim-ply trying to shift the blame to someone else?

At the end of his account he says he has had nightmares about what would have happened to the 'kiddy' if it had gone into the incinera-tor, yet he is not as distressed by imagining what happens during the abortion. Perhaps this is because he does not know exactly what hap-pens, and yet he implies that he does know what they do.

The use of language here could prompt some discussion: what is the effect of using standard English for the doctor and the mother, but forms of the vernacular for the boilerman, the father and the porter? Some readers may see this use of the different forms of speech – dialects and/or idiolects – as no more than naturalism: 'That's just how they would actually speak'. Others might see it as establishing different territories. Finally, some might see even 'naturalism', the attempt to represent things 'as they are', as something that is socially defined, not fixed – a matter of interpretation, again, rather than 'fact'.

The mother's account strikes a strong contrast with the words of the boilerman, partly because of the return to standard English, so that we go from

The Boilerman
An yet ye'd wonder, wid ye no?

to

The Mother
I've no idea who the father is.

There is also a shift in tone, from the boilerman's concern – and perhaps fear – to the mother's apparent lack of concern. Yet she does convey the extent of the problem she, and her mother, have had with her father, and the details of her account, in fact, do convey that her 'I've no idea who the father is' is a literal rather than unconcerned statement.

Her sense of responsibility and guilt, however, does come through at the end of her account. She reveals that she thinks her actions are 'not good' and she explicitly states that she will not try to defend them. The last few lines convey the long-term effects of the events on her: 'I'm sick/ of thinking, regretting, wishing, blaming./ I've gone so dead I see it all/ like pulled from someone else's womb....'

Unlike the mother, the father shows no remorse, but, like her, he has no clear memory of events. He can, however, remember more details than she can. His account contains details of the sex he, and the other two, had with the woman after she had passed out from the effects of drink. He is unperturbed by the news of what might have been his child, and exposes himself as vain and selfish; he remembers that he enjoyed himself.

Finally, the porter seems to have come out of this badly. He seems to have attempted, initially, to absolve himself by denying that he knew the child was still alive. He has clearly benefited from advice from the sheriff and now appears keen, bordering on desperate, to set the record straight. His use of humour, intentionally or not, lightens the tone of the poem at this stage: 'Ah canny go aboot openin disposal bags –/ if ah did ah'd be a nervous wreck'. Yet his repeated, repetitive denial, which brings the poem to a close, conveys his distress: 'Don't answer nothin incriminatin, says the sheriff./ And that's good enough for yours truly./ And neither ah did, neither ah did,/ neither ah did, neither ah did.'

> Is he distressed because he has been subjected to legal interrogations or because he found the child?
> Is he afraid he is going to be blamed?

Each of these accounts gives different insights into events. Each character in this poem also reveals his/her own sense of the rights and wrongs of the situation. The doctor sees himself as clearly in the right and has no need to find fault with anyone else. The boilerman is more outraged at the porter almost becoming a child murderer than he is at the abortions that take place in the hospital. The mother sees herself as very much in the wrong, in spite of seeing her original motivation as both good and bad. The father has no sense that any wrong has been done by himself. The porter sees himself as the most likely scapegoat. That they all have different backgrounds, different experiences and different values is clearly conveyed by the poem.

Like the characters in this poem, participants in our group had different views on the issues raised by this poem. These were identified in a short writing task, where participants could take time to work out their own reactions. A number of specific questions have been raised in this discussion of each section of the poem. A more general question could allow participants more room to develop their own perspectives:

> What is your gut feeling about this case?

or

> What in your view are the rights and wrongs of this case?

In open discussion we began to recognize the power of our personal and professional experiences to shape our views. Yet we also saw a value in defining moral standards for personal and professional life. The hierarchy among professions, and other workers, was seen as a potential danger to moral thinking and action.

In the final phase of our discussion, one group considered that involving non-medical people in ethical decision making would be a healthy development. Some felt that ethical discussions should be more 'front-line', more 'mainstream', rather than taking place in the margins or behind closed doors. There was, finally, some discussion about ways of bringing ethical discussions into other levels, not just leaving the whole ethics agenda to research committees.

Further reflection

During this session we had looked at four different kinds of text, including our own writing. In our discussion we had covered various views and values. We found it useful to conclude our session with 5 minutes' writing to take stock.

The process of looking back at our initial writings, produced at the start of this session, and comparing them with some of the points and arguments raised in our discussion could clarify areas for consolidation on this complex issue, or areas for shifting ground, or the continuing confusion of unresolved issues.

If participants prefer to use prompts for this final writing activity they could generate their own, out of points raised in our discussion, or in their own writing. Here are some examples from our discussion:

What is the basis for judgement in genetic engineering?
Can you see a basis for your judgements in this discussion?
Is there an underlying principle in your interpretations and your writing?
Are your judgements primarily based on

- social justice
- human values
- religious values
- scientific advancement
- the individual's right to choose
- society's right to enforce a general ethical code?

Have you experienced value conflicts in this discussion?

What to do with unresolved issues?

Consider why they are unresolved. Are the questions too wide? Are we unsure of our facts? Do we lack a personal/professional voice in the debate? Have we ourselves failed to understand the broader – i.e. broader than our individual views – social-scientific context? Is the issue so complex – morally – that it is not possible to resolve it, even after reading and discussion? Or is this an issue for which society will not be able to develop guidelines or controls? Is it therefore an issue that even society cannot resolve?

Unresolved issues may be more likely with this topic, since it is so new and covers several branches of science, but other topics may have the same effect. Unresolved issues can be taken forward for future discussions, particularly if further examples or research findings emerge in the academic, literary or popular press.

Why should all the issues be 'resolved'? Is it possible to judge each case of genetic engineering, with assurance, on its own merits? Are there certain underlying principles? Do we have our own set of values and can we apply them here? Are our values still in some way evolving in order to accommodate new developments, new definitions of what it means to be human in genetic engineering terms? Or should certain values be constants? Or is it that we feel a moral obligation to clarify our own moral position, in spite of the complexity – i.e. would **not** taking a stand on this issue be morally acceptable?

If there is a feeling in the group that the issue is unresolved and that this discussion nevertheless needs some closure, some sense of an ending, then perhaps a short writing task here would enable participants to identify a touchstone. This might help participants to individualize, again, their response to genetic engineering. In describing their version of lack of resolution on this issue they may not resolve it for themselves but may, perhaps equally importantly, clarify their own standpoint, however uncertain it may be.

9 Taking stock: *A Little Stranger*

What have we done so far? ● *Taking stock: recurring issues, activities, readings, group processes, professional practice* ● *Questionnaire on the impact of medical humanities* ● *Reactions of different groups* ● *Facilitator's reflections* ● *Forming a new group* ● *Ways of expressing interpretations*

Three 'taking stock' processes are considered in this chapter: firstly, taking stock of the ground covered in this book up to this point; secondly, taking stock of a group's experience of medical humanities after several meetings; and thirdly, taking stock of my own experiences as facilitator of various groups, including one-off groups and the long-running Glasgow group.

In addition, since the primary purposes of this half of the book are to illustrate texts that can be used in medical humanities discussions and to demonstrate how, this chapter follows the pattern of all the chapters in the second half of this book by including a treatment of another literary text.

What have we done so far? The first chapter introduced medical humanities in simple, general and non-threatening terms, outlining its potential purposes and reinforcing what I hope was a positive impression with participants' enthusiastic reactions.

The second chapter provided a step-by-step guide to running a medical humanities discussion, including observed patterns of discussion to help facilitators manage the ebb and flow of narration and reflection.

The third chapter contained an overview of literary and non-literary texts, with brief comments on each, in order to give a flavour of the kinds of thing we say about texts. The diversity of texts was designed to show the abundance of material, rather than to overwhelm the potential facilitator. Some of these texts are dealt with in more detail in the second part of this book.

The fourth chapter gave an overview of methods, including the theme approach, and illustrated a range of issues for discussion, from 'the big issues' to 'daily dilemmas'.

There is a progression in this first half of the book, throughout these four chapters, which is designed to lead the reader from general descriptions and definitions on to more specific illustrations of topics, activities, patterns of discussion, outcomes and feedback from participants. The second half of the book, Chapters 5–8, has therefore been much more detailed, outlining specific discussions we have had in our group about specific texts.

This progression could operate on several levels; there are different challenges in each chapter and in each session, in terms of the readings used, texts, writing activities, levels and kinds of learning, and the potential impact of each discussion on personal and professional lives.

This series of challenges could be defined as a number of stages. Here is one outline of how I see the stages in our group's discussions, which have to a certain extent shaped this sequence of chapters:

- The medical humanities group first learned to be comfortable discussing literary texts, learned a little of the vocabulary for talking about texts and used writing freely to express their own views.
- The group then began to establish a framework, including, for example, initial reflection, discussion and further reflection. The new challenge at this stage lay in the interaction of different views and interpretations, as participants developed confidence in expressing their views.
- Next they focused on one theme, perhaps a difficult theme or a difficult text, so the new challenge at this stage lay in 'puzzling' over the text and using their own questions to move the discussion forward.
- Finally, there was the challenge of moral ambiguity: not only did participants have to tolerate differences of view within the group but they also had to tolerate the feeling of containing different views within themselves. Even at the end of such a discussion they might still feel as if they were being pulled in different directions by different issues or by different cases.

Different groups will presumably experience stages in their work together in different ways; they may move through these stages like our group, but at a different pace. This is not to say that the discussion group moves though a linear process and never looks back; on the contrary, different readings can move participants back and forth in this sequence. Perhaps 'progression of challenges' suggests too strongly a linear hierarchy of tasks.

However, varying the tasks and changing the challenges has been a guiding principle in both the choice of texts and questions for discussion. Creating variety in readings and discussion may require some conscious thinking about pedagogical processes and some design work on the part of the facilitator: **What are the potential learning**

points behind what have loosely been referred to as 'talking points' in this book? Can these be made explicit, without driving the group towards them? Possibly not. Therefore, **is it perhaps better if discussion is genuinely open to all inputs, i.e. genuinely shaped by participants' contributions?** Is it useful not to specify aims and objectives, learning points and challenges but useful from time to time, as now, to take stock of them? These questions could be discussed by members of the group themselves. Personally, my preference – and I think this is the strength of our group – is to allow participants to shape the discussion. This is, in my view, what has kept the discussions stimulating. Moreover, working in this way is in itself challenging.

These questions of progression, planning and impact are the focus for these last two chapters, which aim to provide a structure for continuing debate while continuing to illustrate medical humanities in practice through examples.

Only one specific example of a literary text is presented in this chapter, in order to provide variation from other chapters, which have included more than one text. There is also a return in this chapter to the literary text, leaving out the non-literary. This focus on a single text could, with enough advance warning, encourage participants to read the whole novel, particularly if, as is the case with *A Little Stranger*, the text has only recently been published and is available in paperback. Above all, focusing on a literary text is intended to prevent a drift back to narration, exclusively, and to a purely medical discussion. In focusing on one text we can also review our techniques and tactics for reading and discussing literature.

The extract we used in our discussion comes towards the end of the novel, when the main character appears to be taking stock of her own story, as she has told it in the novel up to this point.

Extract from Candia McWilliam's *A Little Stranger*

The only full description of a work of eating I have served you so far was when I described to you the blue and white bowls of nuts, laid out after supper. Enough to keep ... What is it nannies say? Enough to starve the feeding millions ...
And that was after eating supper....
My hogging began in joy. I was a pig in muck. Not two, not four, but ten of everything. I moved with the times; I was a decimal eater. I believed in eating only the best and I made it beautiful. I contemplated its beauty before commencing engorgement. The virtue of the food, its rarity and cost, the secrecy of its preparation, the hidden expeditions mounted for it, gave my votive sessions the nocturnal glamour of a love affair. By day I cut normal sections from the pies in the larder. By night no moon of cheese could satisfy me....
At its height, the midnight feasting was Dutch, wanting only an urn of tulips to freeze it to still life. I arranged cold fowl (which I ate, wrenching like a midwife with my hands) and sausages with flecks of white fat. On pewter dishes I dumped clouds of bread and flitches of striped speck. Transparent red smoked

beef hung over plates, silky as poppy petals. I tumbled grapes from blue to yellow and the weak purple of primulas. I cushioned myself with Bries rich as white velvet. All this in trencherly quantities.

It was so beautiful; how could it do harm?

At the same time, Margaret was carrying out her inverted worship of the same god....

If it is so that the fat wish to be a shadow of their former selves, the sickly thin wish to be the flesh of their future selves, not a flesh fed by nourishment, but the plump, taut, muscled and yet tender flesh of romance – ready to be carved. While they reject and vomit food, for what are these girls paying, these girls wanting to be hollow? What fantastic connection has been made between daydreams of beauty and romance and that life of bitter spitting?

How I longed to be but a shadow. I had taken myself seriously, but had not at any point taken seriously that self. pp. 127–132

Initial reflection

One option for prompting initial reflective writing is to invite comments on this description:

What is your reaction to this character's way of taking stock of her own story?

Another could be to suggest a focus on a particular word, phrase or detail in the description of food – which proved to be the focal point of the first stage in our discussion in any case. For example, what is the effect of using 'Bries' in the plural?

Readers could pause at this point to consider how they – or you – would put their – your – reaction into words.

Brief discussion, after the 5 minutes' writing and small group discussion, revealed the reactions of the whole group as quite varied: some had quite personal responses to the descriptions, others read between the lines and wondered about the cause of this excess. However much we might have agreed that this person had had – and perhaps still had – a problem with eating, there was still variety in our interpretations, the main points of which are as follows:

Overeating ... compulsive ... no control ...

Not anorexic ... she's big ... or she says she is ...

Could it be some other condition ... or is she not telling us the truth? ...

Excess ... so much of everything ... making it into a ritual ...

Taking pleasure in food ... but intense ...
Sensuous response to food ... sensuous descriptions ...
A hidden pleasure ... solitary ...
Not wanting to take responsibility ... not able to stop ...
Almost taking pride in this ...
Some strange combinations ... is she Dutch? ...
She's very lonely ...
Very plausible ... but not totally credible ...
Threatened by something ... is there jealousy here?

Each of these comments, made by different people in a group of about 16, relate to different parts of the extract. 'Overeating ... compulsive ... no control', for example, is there throughout this extract, from 'hogging' at the start. The initial descriptions, 'Not two, not four, but ten', seem exaggerated, but gradually become more and more convincing, with more and more detail.

The issue of control is interesting, giving the almost ritualistic arrangement of food and eating; yet, there is also the secretiveness. The details of hiding hint at the fact that even this narrative may not be the whole story. We did not feel that this read like a confession; it was more like a display, almost with bravado.

We had some discussion about the specific eating disorder which could be the problem here, sharing our knowledge of different conditions and assessing this woman's condition from the information she gives us. We recognized the role of control, or lack of it, which has been said to be one of the causes of these disorders. The emotional context for her condition also came up in our discussion – we speculated about her having a fear of responsibility or being jealous of someone, possibly Margaret, who is mentioned in this extract. Could she, in fact, be seeking an equal portion of attention here, given that Margaret seems to have had her share? Was Margaret the threat?

We spent so much of our initial reflection phase talking about the descriptions of food and the nature of the problem they concealed, we thought, that we did not really get around to talking about the other question of whether or not this woman is taking stock of her own story, or of her own life. The power of the graphic descriptions to distract us was seen by some as exactly the point: the descriptions provide an elegant and fascinating smoke-screen to some very real problems. Some of the descriptions almost seem to be unlike food: 'I dumped clouds of bread ... I tumbled grapes from blue to yellow and the weak purple of primulas'. In particular, the details of the 'cold fowl (which I ate, wrenching like a midwife with my hands) and sausages with flecks of white fat', were, we found, almost mesmerizing. Those in the group who had worked with midwives found these details particularly distracting. The use of 'Bries', not normally used in the plural, was an effective way of conveying excess.

Having returned to the 'taking stock' question, we realized – yet again – that we would have to define our terms: what does 'taking stock' mean? However, by this time, we had realized that this process of definition was not a mechanical process of checking the dictionary, nor did we expect to agree a common definition among ourselves; instead, we produced several definitions, some of which fitted what this character seemed to be doing and some of which did not.

In some ways, she **is** taking stock, in that she looks back and considers the overall effect of her narrative and identifies a significant omission: 'The only full description of a work of eating I have served you so far was when ...' In another sense, she is almost literally taking stock, as she lists the food she has been eating and the ways in which she has been eating it. Her 'stock' is her food. It could also be her words, since she seems to savour them just as much.

It was on this last point that our answers to the question of taking stock were balanced: still revelling in the excess and in descriptions of it, as she is, we felt that the problem could not yet be resolved. If taking stock implied looking back and moving on – as it did for some in our group – then we were not convinced that taking stock was what she was doing. She was giving a good impression of it, particularly in the last lines of this extract, where she appears to arrive at self-knowledge. But there were some in our group who were not convinced that this was genuine self-knowledge. They could see the character distancing herself from 'these girls' who did have a problem quite like hers, though she does not say this. Moreover, the reflective style here did not, for us, sit well with the excesses of the bulk of the extract. These interpretations raised interesting questions about taking people's – or patients' – stories at face value ... or with a pinch of salt.

Again, there is ambiguity in the text: there is the overt claim to be redressing the balance in her story and the covert attempt to win over the reader: **Is she taking stock or covering up?** This is a question which we could have continued to debate, even on the basis of this short extract.

Discussion for small groups and plenary

In order to give more time to this ambiguity – to explore it further – I offered a question which would focus discussion on the last lines of the extract: 'How I longed to be but a shadow. I had taken myself seriously, but had not at any point taken seriously that self':

Has she begun to take herself seriously now?

Responses to this question varied, from bewilderment to definite answers, both in 'yes' and 'no':

Yes, because she has become aware of her problem.
She seems to have got inside the problem, sees that she hasn't been taking herself seriously and will begin to do so now.
Well, she still feels that she's not good enough.
She still seems to be glorying in the excess of her eating, and she doesn't seem to think that it is a problem in that bit of the story where she describes the food.
We're baffled!
She mixes up personal details and dogmatic statements. It gets a bit disjointed at times.
She has described someone else's illness in more detail than her own, as if distancing herself from her own illness, or distracting us from her problem.
Is it a good thing to take yourself seriously? I know that's not the question, but it would help me to decide.
She shows she understands the mechanics of her problem, but not the psychology. She is very plausible, but can we believe everything she says, either about herself or about the others?
She's nuts!
No. The language is too clever. It doesn't fit. Though she is an intelligent woman, she uses strange words and images to distract us from what is really happening – that she still has a problem and is hiding it.

This selection of comments does not include every response to my question, nor every facet of each response, as it was developed by the individual, since many of these responses were elaborated over several sentences or more. What this selection aims to show is the variety of responses and the range of reasons given for them: some people have been influenced by the style, some are reading the psychology of the woman in terms of their knowledge of eating disorders and others are thinking about causes of the condition. While there is this range of views there also seems to be implicit agreement that this character's words cannot simply be taken at face value.

The text, therefore, is ambiguous, not just because it is open to many interpretations as in the last line of 'After an Operation' – there is also ambiguity in the narrator's own account. Can we trust what she says, even when she appears to be taking us into her confidence? Our group felt, on the whole, that we could not. So our answer to the question is that she may, in a sense, be taking herself seriously but this will not bring self-knowledge and recovery but further denial and illness. In this text, it seems, the ambiguity has not left the text open to interpretation but has in fact shaped our interpretation.

Futher reflection

A final reflective writing activity for this discussion could be to ask participants to think, and write, about the meaning of 'taking stock'. What does it mean? And why do most of us, in spite of the many possible definitions of taking stock, agree that this character is not achieving this?

Given that we will, probably, all define taking stock in different ways, how is it that we have not found one or two definitions which, at least partly, relate to what this character is doing?

This writing activity could bring together a number of phases of this discussion, along with individual readers' views. In addition, the process of defining words will help to open up some of the differences in our assumptions and expectations.

This definition of taking stock should also help to prepare for actually taking stock of medical humanities in the second half of this session, and of this chapter.

Taking stock: recurring issues

At the time of this discussion medical humanities was still quite new to us. We decided to take stock simply by listing and grouping recurring issues in our discussions. Inevitably, this led us to think about why these issues should recur.

Other groups, looking for a prompt for taking stock of their own discussions, could use our list of recurring issues. Alternatively, the facilitator could produce a list of points covered, if s/he has kept notes of the discussions, or members of the group could produce their own lists to initiate a review session. This review could be based on questions that prompt recall rather than evaluation as the first stage:

> What have been the recurring issues for us?
> What questions have we raised in our discussions?
> What are the implications, if any, of our discussions, beyond this group?

The mixture of points and prompts that follows is what we produced in the course of our review session. Some of the issues we recalled from previous discussions raised, for us, further questions for future discussions. Our points are included here both to prompt reflection for others and to guide facilitators by showing the potential outcome of this review. Other groups may produce quite different lists and notes, in quite different forms, and they may find it interesting to compare theirs with ours.

All of our recurring issues have been clustered here into six areas: recovery, 'benchmarks', good practice, objectives and measures, assessment and texts. Within these areas, there is a mixture of ideas, topics, research questions, vague ideas and specific goals, just as we produced them.

One group takes stock: recurring issues in medical humanities

---

What does 'recovery' mean?

What about psychological recovery?
How can we know that it has taken place?
Is there any way to predict who will need help and who will not?
Pre-op behaviours?
What about the involvement of partners: another dimension of the problem of recovery for breast cancer patients?
How can we involve them in 'recovery'?
It has been suggested that all patients, with different kinds of breast cancer, have the same psychological difficulties, especially when thinking about the rest of their lives, their future; how can this help us to help patients recover?

'Benchmarks' and 'milestones'

Pre-op, post-op, post 1 month, post 6 months, post other factors affecting recovery, other 'benchmarks' of recovery (e.g. partner's reactions):
What are the needs of patients at each of these stages?
Can patients – and partners – be involved in setting some of these 'benchmarks' or 'milestones'?

Promoting good practice (rather than 'medic bashing')

From general practice to good practice?: find more examples of good practice and encourage it.

Use cardiac rehab group as an example; patient writings as source of positive feedback.

Will it be more positive about nurses and physios than about doctors?

Would this change if we had more doctors in this group?

Why is it that they do not join us?

Objectives and measures

How do we know that medical humanities has the effects we say it has?

On us only? On students? On staff?

How to measure this effect?:

- Questionnaires
- Profile of mood states (POMS)
- Anxiety scales
- Partner measures
- Patient journals
- Partner journals
- Our journals.

Gather feedback on active participation in recovery:

- Adherence to exercise
- Drugs
- Prescribed treatments or rehab.

What is the objective, in using medical humanities (with patients, staff or students)?:

- Stopping the panic
- Promoting reflection
- Encouraging discussion
- Social interaction.

Are there different objectives when we ask patients to write?:

- Identifying difficult issues
- Facing problems
- Expressing pent-up emotions
- Getting things out of their system
- Anticipating problems.

Assessing students

Different kinds of questions to test awareness in students, not just factual knowledge
Encourage them to give different kinds of answer
Important that assessment includes this kind of activity, otherwise students will not see it as important

- For example, ask physio students to write case notes for stroke patient and for anxious partner, not just for patient
- Allow equal marks for both part of the question and note how much time and detail students devote to each part of the question
- Compare answers of students who have had some medical humanities experience and those who have not
- Would this give some measure of the effect of medical humanities on students' definition of care? (This needs more definition.)

Different texts for different readers?

Need for an annotated reading list?
Which medical humanities texts are useful for patients and which for professionals?
Need to choose carefully?

This summary of our review discussion contains as many questions as statements, which is not unusual for our group, given the lack of consensus and the lack of desire for it. We also produced what are almost action points for future work in medical humanities in order, for example, to be able to measure its effects or to give a better account of its effect on us. This review process also helped us to take one step further forward in calculating the effect of medical humanities or us as individuals and on us as a group.

This activity could be repeated, in order to see which issues concerned a group at different times. This might also reveal the shifting interests of a group over time. Since these ideas are just at the exploratory stage here, it could be important to recycle this list in order to develop some of the ideas and to take stock of those which have progressed between one review and another, those which have resulted in action and of any evaluation of that action.

There are ideas here for moving on in both professional and personal terms and in both academic and clinical contexts. Many of these points, perhaps because of the composition of the group during this session, are concerned with educational processes and making connections; the question of how to connect medical humanities with existing practice in existing structures – and the question of whether or not we should do so – concerned us then and concerns us still. Overall, the themes of our review are as follows:

- making connections within existing infrastructures, rather than standing apart from them;
- addressing specific questions about clinical practice;
- finding a theoretical base e.g. reflective practice;
- continuing to accommodate differences;
- evaluating reflection.

This summary of issues and questions raised by our group could be used as memory jogger for other groups, prior to them carrying out an evaluation of their own group. Individuals could take stock using questions developed by the facilitator or by the group, as in Chapter 1, where selected responses were included.

> **Taking stock: activities, readings, group processes and professional practice**

In our evaluation we used the following questions in order to review activities, readings and group processes, putting one question on an A4 page in order to allow participants plenty of room to write their responses.

Questionnaire

> **What did you think of 'literature' before you first came along to this group?**
>
> What thoughts and feelings did you associate with the word 'literature'? What experience had you had of literature? What was your view of its usefulness?

> **Have you changed any of these views since then?**
>
> Has working in this group confirmed or altered – or a bit of both – these views? Has your attitude to literature changed? Have you revised your definition of 'literature'? Or has it remained pretty much the same as it was before?

> **Have your group work skills developed as a result of working in this group?**
>
> – e.g. speaking, listening, debating, keeping to the point, or any other skills?

> **Has your attitude to writing – i.e. doing some writing – changed as a result of working in this group?**
>
> Do you think about it differently? Do you see it as having a different role or use in your life or work?
>
> **Has being in this group affected how you teach and/or do your job?**

I wrote these questions in order to get a general view of what people thought about medical humanities after 2 years of discussions, meeting every 6–8 weeks. I tried to keep the questions informal and hoped that leaving a lot of empty space on each page would encourage participants to write freely. I distributed the questionnaire towards the end of a session and participants posted it back to me.

The main purpose, therefore, was to give participants time to reflect for themselves. A secondary purpose was to capture snapshots or a synthesis of these reflections in evaluating the work of the whole group. I was also looking for information on what skills they thought they had developed in literary analysis.

Since I frequently did not participate in discussions at that time, this was participants' opportunity to 'speak' directly to me.

In addition, reflection on group processes could be explored in more detail, with open questions about what the participants think the group processes have been; i.e. asking them simply to describe the group processes:

How would you describe our way of working together as a group?
What role(s) has the facilitator played?

Answers to these two questions could be quite wide-ranging, across a group. Sharing these answers, in pairs, twos and fours, might prove very interesting. My own description of our group processes in this book, for example, have prompted a few participants who read these chapters in draft form to say 'Oh, so that's what we've been doing!', which implies, to me, that their version could be different.

More specific questions could focus on the role of participants in the group process. Not all participants will feel comfortable with these questions. Some will already have given them some thought; others will not.

What do you feel you have contributed to the group?
What do you feel the group has given you?
What role do you usually find yourself playing in group?
What role have you played in this group; e.g. have you found yourself participating in discussions in particular ways? Have you interacted with others, including the facilitator, in particular ways?

Changes in group processes may have been observed by participants and it may be important to put observations in context, particularly since membership of the group is not constant:

> Have you observed any changes in the way we have worked together as a group?

The main point here is to stress the value of observations, without judgements at this stage. The process of recalling and expressing observations to each other can become here part of the group process, or group 'maintenance'. This discussion could usefully shift some of the responsibility for the culture of the group from the facilitator and back to the participants.

Reactions of different groups

Responses to these questions by participants in our mixed group are illustrated in Chapter 1. They were very positive.

The responses of the long-running group make interesting comparisons with the responses of other groups participating in one-off sessions. Over the past 7 years I have given introductory sessions on medical humanities to many different groups:

- **Physiotherapists**: national and international conferences
- **Nurses**: conferences and students
- **Podiatrists**: students
- **Humanities**: PhD students
- **Scottish literature**: international summer school students
- **Clinical reasoning**: postgraduates
- **Roadshow groups**: post-qualification physiotherapists, nurses, medics
- **University lecturers**: Teaching and Learning in Higher Education course
- **Women's studies**: lecturers and postgraduates

Physiotherapists at national and international conferences have tended to react most positively, if active participation and enthusiasm for medical humanities can be taken as measures of positive reactions. Most groups have reacted positively once they have got over the initial fear of 'literature'.

However, some groups – a minority – have been more reticent, including, surprisingly, PhD students in humanities. I expected that, of all of these groups, the humanities students, particularly those in English Literature, would be the most likely to be interested in medical humanities. I did find that one group of international summer school students and their lecturers saw medical humanities as a new and exciting approach to literature. However, the postgraduate humanities group were slow to engage in the process of discussion and quick to question its theoretical basis and practical purpose.

This was interesting; each group, of course, brings new questions to their first experience of medical humanities. What was even more interesting was that I had used the same poem with them that I had used on the medical humanities roadshow: 'After an Operation'. In all the roadshow groups this poem provoked instant and prolonged discussion, using the structure outlined in these chapters; the postgraduate humanities group, by contrast, needed more encouragement to get started and keep going in their discussion. One of them commented that they were not used to being asked to have discussions in their seminars, and this might have been part of the response to the way I introduced medical humanities, which is always participative at some stage.

They seemed uncomfortable with the open agenda we use in our medical humanities group, with our lack of attention to the theoretical basis of what we are doing.

This seminar and the valuable questions raised by this group was another reminder to me of the difficulty of moving out of the territory of the discipline; what I mean by that is that I expected these students to feel quite at home with the idea of discussing a poem. I had forgotten that they might have some difficulty with **our approach** to discussing poems. I had forgotten that our approach is different, in some ways, from how it is approached in literature, sociology or other humanities departments. And yet, our approach is only different in some ways.

I continued this session using the structure of reflective writing and talking that has evolved in our group work, but left plenty of time for questions about medical humanities – rather than about the text and their writings – since this was what people wanted to discuss.

Working with this group raised a question, for me, about flexibility: are there some groups who cannot be, or who take longer to become, flexible in their approach to their subject? This takes me back to an earlier question raised in an earlier chapter: does specializing in a subject inevitably lead to a narrow focus? Are specialists able or willing to bridge the gaps between their specialisms? Yet reluctance to cross disciplinary boundaries cannot be the whole story, since some of the postgraduate group were doing PhDs that crossed disciplinary boundaries.

An even more interdisciplinary group – of Women's Studies students and lecturers – were much more open in discussion and apparently more flexible in their approach. Perhaps the difference is that they did not bring to the discussion a purely – i.e. solely – literary response. In their responses they themselves drew on or referred to several different disciplines and to their own experience.

Facilitator's reflections

Was it just me? Did I just do a less stimulating session? Or are some groups not as ready to talk about literature in a variety of ways? Is this why they were uncomfortable with the medical humanities aim of including varieties of response, i.e. **any** response, not just 'legitimate' responses within a certain range? I myself am developing an uncomfortable feeling that specialisms have a tendency to 'territorialism' and that people who see themselves as specialists sometimes, not always, have a need to defend the territory of their specialism. This may apply – I am speculating now – to other kinds of specialists and other professions, including the medical and health professions. I am speculating in this way because I find myself struggling to accept the possibility that this postgraduate group were **unable** to discuss the poem. But I realize that there may also be an element of truth here – perhaps their group skills are different from, or less developed than, what I expected.

What does all this add up to? This summary of my post-seminar reflections is included here for two reasons. My first reason is to extend the debate about the place of medical humanities in existing structures and systems, like, for example, the curriculum for undergraduate students and the programme for continuing professional development. The question here is where does medical humanities fit? – our group sits outside of existing structures. There is also the question of how does it fit? – how can the value of this new approach be made to fit an existing professional value system?

My second reason for including my reflections here is to give potential facilitators a few insights into my own experiences in a variety of contexts. I have deliberately included both positive and negative experiences and suggested one or two strategies for maintaining dialogue.

What the experience of talking to these diverse groups has taught me is that different versions of the medical humanities approach could be developed with different groups. This very obvious learning point should, it will no doubt be observed, have hit me somewhat earlier and at several hundred miles an hour, given that one of the goals of medical humanities is to help people to find their own route into the discussion. However, perhaps different questions are needed to prompt discussion. This question of differences in approaches for different groups had also, interestingly, cropped up in our review of recurring issues summarized above.

Differences in reactions across groups, which might be brought out in discussion of group processes, might raise questions about differences in group processes. In taking stock, in these reflections, and thinking ahead to new groups, there are four questions which sum up my points while keeping the issues open for others:

> Do these different groups have different group processes?
> Do they need different questions to prompt discussion?
> Can they use medical humanities in different ways?
> Do they bring different purposes to medical humanities discussions?

Perhaps the facilitator has to be ready to play a different role. Perhaps the group has to be encouraged to explore some of the value judgements that are made by one discipline of another; for example, doctors have been known to make certain value judgements about nurses and physiotherapists and occupational therapists have been known to enjoy, if that is the right word, a similar relationship.

The politics of these relationships is perhaps a factor here. Some professional groups value the language and rhetoric of their own discipline so highly that it is difficult for them to value any other; interacting with the rhetoric of other disciplines is genuinely difficult.

My own 'taking stock' on working with different groups has raised, for me, questions about the implications of what I see as a language barrier between professions:

> How does this language barrier affect relationships within the health-care team?
> Is this what makes it difficult to build bridges between the different professional groups in the health-care team?
> Could medical humanities be useful in counteracting what I see as 'territorialism'?
> Could medical humanities be useful as a diagnostic process, at the start of a learning process, since it so quickly reveals the ways in which people are thinking and the extent to which they are ready to think differently?

Medical humanities has proven itself to be one of the few places where the health professions can have a genuine dialogue; anyone managing or participating in medical humanities will presumably have to find a way around this language barrier. What is it about the Glasgow group, the group I have worked with most, which has

allowed this barrier to be broken down? Perhaps it has been our deliberately experimental approach – 'let's try this' – and letting the group
shape discussions even when they were not sure of what to say.
Perhaps this very positive group effect depends on the group management skills of the facilitator; constructive feedback from participants on my group management skills have forced me to acknowledge
my own role in this group effect. Yet I feel I myself am always learning
in the group and always 'playing it by ear', never sure in advance of
how people will react or what they will say. In fact, I am never quite
sure in advance what role I am going to play. With any new group I
always expect to learn something, not just about them or about the
subject but about my own approaches and assumptions.

Forming a new group

What would get a new group off to a good start? Someone from our
group could start up and/or support a new group. Having someone in
the group who has already had some experience of medical humanities would perhaps give participants and facilitators the confidence
that they could keep the discussion going. Someone who has been in
a medical humanities group over several years will, moreover, have
developed skills in literary analysis and group discussion.

Since this is not going to be feasible for everyone who wants to set
up a new group, it is a good strategy to have one or two people who
are very interested in the idea of medical humanities and who will
become the core group who can keep it going. Building the group
around a core of like-minded people implies targeting people initially
who are likely to be interested. One or two could share the responsibility of facilitating.

It is also constructive to have people who are **not** like-minded, even
sceptical, in at the start, since any effective group has to learn to allow
space and voice for varieties of views. To find that we reached a consensus in our views on complex issues and having read texts that are
inherently open to multiple interpretations would be cosy but then
boring and ultimately troubling. Such people may have responded to
the advert about the first meeting, for example, and may need particular encouragement, since they may have recognized that they are not
'like-minded' with the targeted core group.

'Take the plunge' with a bit of confidence and interest in the
approach, without too much in the way of an agenda, without too
high an expectation of the first few meetings, without worrying too
much about the purpose of it all and, perhaps most importantly, not

forgetting to provide decent coffee and maybe even some biscuits, to keep things relatively informal. Having the expectation that the new medical humanities group will be as enjoyable and stimulating as ours, and being able to convey this to others, could help to break the ice.

This text can be mined for ideas, readings and prompts for writing and discussion. Topics that have worked in our discussion can be used for other discussions. There are questions here which have been effective in stimulating debate. Using the texts included in this book could provide a framework for discussion and a safety net for facilitators.

What I have learned from my work with various groups is that working with physiotherapists or including some in the group along with nurses and non-medical people is likely to be successful in getting the group started. I would be happy to be proved wrong here, but it is my experience that they are more receptive and more discursive, particularly a post-qualification group like ours. Also, anyone who is interested in interdisciplinary work could be persuaded to attend a meeting or two. In fact, it is in an attempt to attract a variety of participants that we vary the venues for meetings, to include hospitals, clinics, conference centres, classrooms, universities and colleges; i.e. we have deliberately chosen clinics and classrooms and non-medical venues.

Flexibility, finally, is one of the key principles, so that our combination of people should all feel that they can have a say in how the group is run and what we read. Our approach of 'give it a go' and 'anything goes' has not, however, left us oblivious to the fact that people need time to develop confidence, to get to know each other, to find their place in the group and to recover the ability to enjoy reading literature for their own interest rather than to pass an exam.

Ways of expressing interpretations

While participants have throughout our work, and in this book, been encouraged to use their own language to articulate their own interpretations of literary texts, occasionally they do ask for help with language they can use. A particular challenge for people who do not have a literary background or training is finding words to distinguish between narration and interpretation. The past tense which they use to talk about what they have experienced has to be distinguished from the present tense they use to talk about what the text suggests.

In addition, specific words should clearly signal whether the speaker is telling us about experience or interpretations: a word like 'experienced' can be used to describe something that has actually happened, while a word like 'suggests' can be used to put into words what the text says to them. For example:

A language for interpreting, using words which signal you are interpreting:

This suggests ...
This conveys ...
This seems to imply ...
One interpretation of this could be ....

Locating your interpretation in the text

Locating the text in a context:

What are the meanings and associations of a word in its present context?
In what context was the text produced: intended reader and purpose?

The point here is to make it clear that we are interpreting by using words which show this, the simplest way being to use the word 'interpret'. The aim is to present an interpretation **as an interpretation**. When we shift from factual statements, for example, to interpretative statements, without this kind of explicit marker, the distinction between narration and reflection may be unclear.

These words can show that the participant's statement is clearly interpretation, either an interpretation in the making, in the form of thinking aloud, or a view which has been developed. While narration and reflection may be closely interwoven for a speaker, and both have been observed in medical humanities discussions, listeners will be able to identify which is which and are more likely to respond appropriately if the speaker has signalled which is which.

The purpose of this chapter was to take stock, or rather to indicate how a group might do so. Reflections from one facilitator are also included. This process of taking stock has involved looking back over activities, readings, group processes and the impact, if there is any, on professional practice. In this way, whatever appears to have become routine for the group can be opened up to the various views of all participants. There may be no group consensus here either. Having done this, however, a group may be ready to 'move on', the subject of the final chapter of this book.

10 Moving on: *Awakenings*

Talking and writing about science: personal, popular and academic ●
Scientific knowledge and literary knowledge ● *'Fact' and 'fiction'* ●
Education: activities and the curriculum ● *Reflective practice* ● *Territorialism*

This concluding chapter considers 'moving on' in two senses:

> How does a medical humanities group move on from here?
> Is scientific writing moving on?

The first question is designed to follow up on the taking stock process covered in the previous chapter by exploring different routes for development. Alternatively, a group could use some of our questions – or their own – to consider how they might move on in their own way. Above all, having taken stock, perhaps periodically, I am suggesting that it can be productive to consider options for future discussions, so that topics and discussions do not become routine. Since the Glasgow group has been successful in attracting participants for over 7 years, I will continue to refer to our own experience for examples, while also opening up other options, since ours is surely not the **only** way to 'do medical humanities'.

The second question is designed to move discussion beyond a strict separation of literary and non-literary texts. The point here is to illustrate a kind of text that is both scientific and non-scientific, in the sense that it deals with a science subject, including scientific presentation of data in some cases, but is written in a different style. In some instances the authors have explicitly challenged the conventions of scientific writing and even the scientific method itself. The result is a creative approach to science, which takes elements of scientific thinking and writing and brings them together with elements of thinking and writing more often found in the humanities.

This chapter, therefore, invites participants explicitly to think not only about the future of the group, but also to rethink assumptions about what constitutes a scientific text.

Initial reflection

Reflective writing could initially focus on the process of moving on:

What does 'moving on' mean?
Do we need to move on in this group?
Do we need to consider this question?

Unlike previous questions for initial writing, these questions may prompt participants to question the question; the group may be very comfortable with the role the facilitator is playing for them and with the questions s/he has produced for them. They may also have focused on their own questions in their own writing – there is always that option. However, encouraging participants explicitly to question the facilitator's question could be one way of moving a group on, and could prevent them from becoming passive recipients of the facilitator's prompts. Inviting participants to question the questions, or responding positively when they do so without an invitation, has been one way of actively involving them in the running of the group and the shaping of its discussions.

Moving on could mean moving to new activities or consolidating what we have developed. It could mean adapting some aspect of our discussion; for example, in our group we decided to fix dates for meetings for the whole year in advance in order to give those who needed more notice a better chance of attending. We also decided to hold all the meetings in the same place, to make it easier for people to find their way there, rather than having to find their way through a different building at each meeting. Moving on could also mean stopping the group and moving on to other activities; in our group, since people tended to drift in and out, sometimes with a break of several months, participants always have had the option to drop in and out as they choose. But there has always been a group who wanted to attend and some who wanted to but could not, because of travelling time or a clash of commitments or childcare responsibilities. Recently, we have moved on in another way by having a half-day Saturday seminar in order to open the group up to new members.

Discussion

This section includes readings and comments which aim to illustrate alternative forms of scientific writing. For discussion, these can be taken individually or together and an underlying question for each is how scientific is this text?

There are six readings in this section. Each of the extracts is shorter than the extract we used for our discussions, but these should nevertheless give a clear idea of the kind of text that seems to be bridging the gap between scientific and non-scientific writing:

1. *Awakenings*, O. Sachs
2. *The Limits of Science*, P. Medawar
3. *Could it be Stress?*, C. Macdonald
4. *Narrative Means to Therapeutic Ends*, M. White and D. Epstein
5. *Illness as Metaphor*, S. Sontag
6. *Able Lives: Women's Experience of Paralysis*, ed. J. Morris.

The first of these, Oliver Sachs's *Awakenings*, is one of those that explicitly challenge the nature of scientific writing and the scientific method.

Extract from Oliver Sachs's *Awakenings*

The theme of this book is the lives and reactions of certain patients in a unique situation – and the implications which these hold out for medicine and science. These patients are among the few survivors of the great sleeping-sickness epidemic (*encephalitis lethargica*) of fifty years ago, and their reactions are those brought about by a remarkable new 'awakening' drug (laevodihydroxy-phenylalanine, or L-DOPA)....

The general style of this book – with its alternation of narrative and reflection, its proliferation of images and metaphors, its remarks, repetitions, asides and footnotes – is one which I have been impelled towards by the very nature of the subject-matter. My aim is not to make a system, or to see patients as systems, but to picture a world, a variety of worlds – the landscapes of being in which these patients reside. And the picturing of worlds requires not a static and systematic formulation, but an active exploration of images and views, a continual jumping-about and imaginative **movement**....

Running throughout this book is a metaphysical theme – the notion that it is insufficient to consider disease in purely mechanical or chemical terms; that it must be considered equally in biological or metaphysical terms, i.e. in terms of organization and design. In my first book, *Migraine*, I suggested the necessity of such a double approach, and in the present work I develop this theme is much greater detail. Such a notion is far from new – it was understood very clearly in classical medicine. In present-day medicine, by contrast, there is an almost exclusively technical or mechanical emphasis, which has led to immense advances, but also to intellectual regression, and a lack of proper attention to the full needs and feelings of patients.   pp. xvii–xviii

Like Malcolm in *Jurassic Park*, Sachs (in his 1973 introduction) not only felt constrained by what he saw as an 'exclusively technical or mechanical emphasis' but also felt the need to work and write in completely different ways, using aspects of style that are often found only in the humanities: 'images ... metaphors ... remarks, repetitions, asides ... active exploration of images of views, a continual jumping-about and imaginative *movement*' (p. xviii). Later, in his introduction to the 1990 edition of *Awakenings*, Sachs referred to another writer who had influenced, if not liberated, him with a combination of 'intellectual power and human warmth' (p. xxxvi), a combination which he had, he said, rarely encountered. For Sachs, this author, A. R. Luria, provided 'an antidote to certain trends in medical writing, which attempted to delete both subjectivity and reflection' (p. xxxvi). Sachs was concerned to include 'subjectivity and reflection' through 'detailed and non-reductive narratives', which he saw not only as a means to describe patients, but also as a means to understand them (p. xxxvii).

Varieties of writings are, in fact, included in Sachs's account of his methods and his findings: scientific data, the writings of philosophers, scientific findings, literary parallels and patients' views. It was an explicit goal to capture the patients' experience of their illness, to capture their subjectivity, not just to express his own. This combination of kinds of information, kinds of thinking and kinds of writing makes for a very rich account of the illness and its treatment. His account seems like an early form of what is now called grounded theory, combining qualitative and quantitative research methods and developing a new way of communicating the outcome of this new hybrid. He even had to find a new name for his cases, and referred to them not just as 'case histories' but also as 'stories' (p. xxxi).

The distinction between scientific and non-scientific writing is quite clear to Sachs. The implications of this distinction, however, seemed to him sufficiently serious that he had to do something about it. His choice of writing in the first person in these introductions makes it very clear that this is his personal view. Yet, he does put this personal view in a context which medical humanities readers will recognize:

I was always conscious of this double need, and found there were always **two** books, potentially, demanded by every clinical experience: one more purely 'medical' or 'classical' – an objective description of disorders, mechanisms, syndromes; the other more existential and personal – an empathic entering into patients' experiences and words.   p. xxxvi

What medical humanities has been striving to do – bring scientific and non-scientific thinking and talking into one discussion – appears to happen in this book, therefore, because this is exactly what Sachs is trying to achieve. This is one example of a text which has moved beyond the divide between science and the humanities. Not that this is a literary text. Not that this undermines the value of discussing literary texts on medical subjects. Sachs's writing validates bringing the humanities closer to the medical context than simply playing a complementary role. Moreover, he has given the skills and approaches of the humanities certain specific functions in the medical context.

Like Sachs, Peter Medawar, in his book *The Limits of Science*, questions what has been called 'the scientific method' (p. 51). His essay 'Can Scientific Discovery be Premeditated?' is a text which I have used to initiate discussion in a third-year undergraduate physics course on Technical Writing. This discussion began to reveal the students' assumptions about scientific methods and scientific writing. The aim of this discussion was to start the students off on the process of considering options for writing – beyond the lab-report formula – to consider writing about their scientific work in a variety of ways and for a variety of audiences, as they would have to after graduation. Medawar's essay deals specifically with the subject of methodology:

Extract from Peter Medawar's *The Limits of Science*

Administrative high-ups in Washington and Whitehall firmly believe that scientists make their discoveries by the application of a procedure known to them as the scientific method – the belief in which, considered as a kind of calculus of discovery, is based on a misconception dating from the days of John Stuart Mill's *A System of Logic* and Karl Pearson's *The Grammar of Science*.

If such a method existed, none of us working scientists would be secure in our jobs, for consider a research worker in an institute devoted to elucidating the causes of and finding a cure for rheumatoid arthritis. If he fails to do so, his failure could only be either because he did not know the scientific method, in which case he should be sacked, or because he was too lazy or obstinate to apply it, an equally valid reason for dismissal.

There is indeed no such thing as 'the' scientific method. A scientist uses a very great variety of exploratory stratagems, and although a scientist has a certain address to his problems – a certain way of going about things that is more likely to bring success than the gropings of an amateur – he uses no procedure of discovery that can be logically scripted. According to Popper's methodology, every recognition of a truth is preceded by an imaginative preconception of what the truth might be – by hypotheses such as William Whewell first called 'happy guesses', until, as if recollecting that he was Master of Trinity, he wrote 'felicitous strokes of inventive talent'.

Most of the day-to-day business of science consists in making observations or experiments designed to find out whether this imagined world of our hypotheses corresponds to the real one. An act of imagination, a speculative adventure, thus underlies every improvement of natural knowledge.   p. 51

Medawar's description of scientific method as 'exploratory strata-gems ... imaginative preconception ... act of imagination, a speculative adventure' blurs the distinction between rational and imaginative thinking in a way that makes the distinction itself seem irrational. Examples of scientific discovery give his argument in this essay added weight; they do indeed illustrate the combination of what he calls 'pre-paredness of mind' and 'exertion and reflection' (p. 50). He also finds a place for his argument in the history and philosophy of science; his frame of reference includes Thomas Kuhn, Karl Popper, John Stuart Mill and Karl Pearson.

Again, the narrow definition of 'scientific method' is questioned. The imagination does have a place in scientific work. The apparent gap between science and humanities is bridged again, in a different way: not so much by using skills and styles of thinking and writing in the humanities to develop a completely different scientific tech-nique, as in Sachs, but by showing the role of imagination in what are usually taken to be more conventional versions of the scientific method, in discoveries that are generally accepted as standard, rather than deviant, as Sachs was judged to be, within the scientific com-munity.

Cameron Macdonald, like Sachs and Medawar, similarly identifies as a weakness, in his book *Could it be Stress?*, the conventional medical method that excludes 'the emotional factors' (p. 76), and sees this exclusion as the cause of confusion in scientific publications on a cer-tain condition:

Extract from Cameron Macdonald's *Could it be Stress?: Reflections on Psychosomatic Illness*

A great deal of published work is available on normal and abnormal water metabolism, and it is characterized by confusing and contradictory statements partly, I suspect, because the emotional factors tend to be ignored. In the stan-dard works, only De Wardener (20) appears to note that stress may produce either diuresis or anti-diuresis....

Dr Glen and I felt we might have a psychosomatic disorder which could be mea-sured (24). We examined a large series of water-retainers and ended up with 55 patients and we used 21 lab workers and medical students as controls. The water retention patients had a significantly lower solute output for the same urine flow compared to the controls ($p = 0.01$). A psychotherapeutic interview tended to increase the solute output and to reduce this difference from the control in the two hours following interview, though not to statistical significance (25)....

On the whole we confirmed the findings of previous workers that situations of stress involving anger, defence and resentment in which the patients tended to withdraw seemed to produce oliguria, while relaxed and reassuring attitudes with easy communication produced an outgoing situation symbolic even in terms of urinary outflow. It seems likely that ordinary healthy people have these

responses also, but do not react with the violent fluctuations which characterize patients with water retention syndromes....

The case histories noted earlier are fairly typical and demonstrate how rapidly
many patients respond to the most ordinary opportunity for sympathetic listening. Certainly many are quite dramatic in their response. One elderly lady with
quite gross oedema attended an outpatient clinic, and when no obvious reason for her fluid retention was found, her immediate family history was scruti-
nized and she reported that her husband was dying of cancer in a surgical
ward at the hospital. While we discussed this sad tale she asked if she might
be excused to empty her bladder so we measured the volume which proved to
be over a litre.   pp. 76, 78–80

Again, scientific data – the usual scientific method and the usual
comparisons – are combined with an assessment of the emotional state
of patients. The association of certain conditions with certain emotions
has, for Macdonald, implications for treatment, but 'treatment' in the
sense of treating the patient in a way that will allow them to express,
rather than repress, their emotions: 'many patients respond to the
most ordinary opportunity for sympathetic listening' (p. 80). That
Macdonald has found that these cases and their responses are 'fairly
typical' adds weight to his argument.

There will be questions here about whether or not health professionals are trained to help patients express and cope with their own
emotions; there will also be questions of whether or not conditions
should be treated without attending to the emotions. Different health
professionals – and scientists – will doubtless have different reactions
to these case histories.

The use of the first person – 'I' – and of personal experience as a
physician, reveals the process of working through a problem in narratives about patients. The physician, in this example, draws on extensive experience, collaborating with colleagues, 'sympathetic listening'
(p. 80) and observations of how patients recover and holds all of this
in the context of the limits of his own knowledge and the limits of scientific knowledge as a whole. In fact, acknowledging limits and con-
tradictions in the knowledge base on this particular condition was his
starting point and his purpose in making his own observations and
using his own judgement.

Far from the rational, systematic model of treating the condition,
this physician has attempted to treat the patient who has the condition. His conclusions to this chapter in his book emphasize the power
of emotions to create the condition:

To summarize – we are as yet ignorant of the exact metabolic pathways that
lead to water retention but in psychotherapy we have a powerful and effective
tool to help recovery in many patients. A typical patient will have been brought
up to repress grief and to avoid weeping. The symptoms arise in situations of
bereavement often associated with guilt.   p. 82

This writing shows the significance of patients' experience, not simply as a background to illness but as a cause of it. Macdonald has argued that treatment must address this cause. The medical condition, he argues, has to be treated in an appropriate way, and perhaps not in a conventional medical way at all. This raises questions of how appropriate it is to write up cases in a conventional medical way. Macdonald's style – of combining 'hard' scientific data with 'soft' human data – provides another example of how the two can be brought together to make a convincing, to me, medical argument.

Story telling – telling the story of a bereavement – was one factor, Macdonald argued, in effective treatment of patients suffering from 'gross oedema' (p. 80). A more detailed account of this strategy, and perhaps a more developed form of this strategy, is provided by White and Epstein in their book *Narrative Means to Therapeutic Ends*:

Extract from M. White and D. Epstein's *Narrative Means to Therapeutic Ends*

Storied therapy
Practice
A therapy situated within the context of the narrative mode of thought would take a form that:

1. privileges the person's lived experience;
2. encourages a perception of a changing world through the plotting or linking of lived experience through the temporal dimension;
3. invokes the subjunctive mood in the triggering of presuppositions, the establishment of implicit meaning, and in the generation of multiple perspective;
4. encourages polysemy and the use of ordinary, poetic and picturesque language in the description of experience and in the endeavour to construct new stories;
5. invites a reflexive posture and an appreciation on one's participation in interpretive acts;
6. encourages a sense of authorship and re-authorship of one's life and relationships in the telling and retelling of one's story;
7. acknowledges that stories are co-produced and endeavours to establish conditions under which the 'subject' becomes the privileged author;
8. consistently inserts the pronouns 'I' and 'you' in the description of events.

p. 83

Certain features of our private writing, in our medical humanities group, are here: the freedom to write about our own experience, to choose to write about a specific question or to brainstorm, the freedom to write about our own perceptions, the freedom to speculate and to write in the first person. We have used a variation of this to explore, in writing, fantasies and possibilities for future actions in an exercise derived from White and Epstein's 'storied therapy':

> If you had a month off – no work, no commitments – what would
> you do? What would you change? What would you keep the
> same? Would you do anything new? Or would you stay on famil-
> iar ground? Would it lead to any changes in your life? You don't
> need to worry about readers; focus on your own notions.
>
> Use words that you would not normally use, even if you are
> unsure of exactly what they mean, or of whether you have used
> them in the right way – in fact, especially if you are not sure that
> you are using them correctly. This also applies to grammar, punc-
> tuation, spelling and handwriting – they are not important here.
> Use different kinds of words and sentences, simple and complex,
> short and long, ordinary and extraordinary. You do not need to
> stick to one idea; you can change your mind half-way through,
> for example, if you want to.
>
> This writing is for discussion only, and you can decide how much
> to say about it. No one will read it unless you want them to, but
> you will have time to talk about what you wrote and about your
> feelings about writing in this way. Write for 15 minutes. Start with
> the sentence 'If I had a month off I would ...'

This writing task was designed to stimulate imaginative writing
while revealing, possibly, needs and desires. Participants were also
encouraged to use words they did not usually use, in order to put into
practice number four in White and Epstein's list, to push the writing
beyond the everyday lived experience to an imagined one.

As with all our writings, these were private and so it is not possible
to reveal what participants wrote. The intended outcome was that participants would use variety in their language and ideas in their own
writing. I felt it was important, in the midst of debate about other people's writings and their various forms and versions of scientific and
medical writing, to give people time to explore, and push against, the
limits of their own writing. This could also, I hoped, be useful in moving us beyond the routines of our own writing in the 5 minutes' writing activities.

There was potential for a number of different outcomes in this writing task and presumably each participant responded to the task in
their own way, with their own emphasis on one or other of my idea of
outcomes.

White and Epstein's text provided plenty of ideas for writing and
reading narratives in therapeutic ways. In the past, participants in our
group had said that they found some of the writing activities we used
'therapeutic', perhaps in a different sense ... but perhaps not.

   This particular writing task illustrated a method for 'moving on' in our own thinking and in our writing: moving on from reflecting on other people's writing, moving on from reflecting on our own experience and moving on from the way we usually write. Of course, although this is a form of fantasy writing, it might, in the process, prompt us to reflect on our present position. In the context of this chapter, therefore, it could provide a mechanism for moving on in both thinking and writing.

   The element of fantasy in this writing task is not as far-fetched or as far-removed from the medical context as it may seem, in that fantasy also has a role in our experience; we respond imaginatively to illness just as we respond imaginatively to other experiences. This process has been described – on an international scale – by Susan Sontag, in her book *Illness as Metaphor* (and the follow-up *Aids as Metaphor*):

Extract from Susan Sontag's *Illness as Metaphor*

I want to describe, not what it is really like to emigrate to the kingdom of the ill and live there, but the punitive or sentimental fantasies concocted about that situation: not real geography, but stereotypes of national character. My subject is not physical illness itself but the uses of illness as a figure or metaphor. My point is that illness is **not** a metaphor, and that the most truthful way of regarding illness – and the healthiest way of being ill – is one most purified of, most resistant to, metaphoric thinking. Yet it is hardly possible to take up one's residence in the kingdom of the ill unprejudiced by the lurid metaphors with which it has been landscaped. It is towards an elucidation of those metaphors, and a liberation from them, that I dedicate this enquiry.

Chapter 1

Two diseases have been spectacularly, and similarly, encumbered by the trappings of metaphor: tuberculosis and cancer.

The fantasies inspired by TB in the last century, by cancer now, are responses to a disease thought to be intractable and capricious – that is, a disease not understood – in an era in which medicine's central premise is that all diseases can be cured. Such a disease is, by definition, mysterious. For as long as its cause was not understood and the ministrations of doctors remained so ineffective, TB was thought to be an insidious, implacable theft of a life. Now it is cancer's turn to be the disease that doesn't knock before it enters ... a role it will keep until, one day, its aetiology becomes as clear and its treatment as effective as those of TB have become.

Although the way in which disease mystifies is set against a backdrop of new expectations, the disease itself (once TB, cancer today) arouses thoroughly old-fashioned kinds of dread. Any disease that is treated as a mystery and acutely enough feared will be felt to be morally, if not literally, contagious. Thus, a surprisingly large number of people with cancer find themselves being shunned by relatives and friends and are the objects of practices of decontamination by members of their household, as if cancer, like TB, were an infectious disease.   pp. 7–10

Sontag argues that it is because we do not understand these particular illnesses that we 'concoct' fantasies about them. She further argues that while not understanding them might be considered quite normal, it is because we expect medicine to cure all ills that we find these illnesses so frightening; that medicine cannot control them is threatening to any expectation that it could.

This kind of writing points out the ways in which representations of illness are created and perhaps make us more conscious of how we express our representations of illness. Usually, medical language aspires to the very liberation from metaphor that Sontag advocates, yet non-medical people, being less likely to use medical language, have to find some way to put into words what's happening to them. The interaction of these languages – the medical and the metaphorical – is where, again, a gap can open up in communications about illness.

We used this text as a starting point for discussions about representations of illness. I took several of Sontag's points and developed some questions to prompt discussion:

Suggested issues for discussion on Sontag's *Illness as Metaphor*

How do we represent disease?

What language do we use?
How should we represent specific diseases and illnesses?
Are there diseases which we need to 'de-mythicize'?

Are diseases 'mystified' by the language we use – as patients and as carers – to describe them?

Do we have to work against/with clichés about illnesses?
'Labels', 'names' and 'index tabs' – how can we write them so that patients can both understand and cope with them?

What are the associations of different diseases?

Cardiac disease? – 'Cardiac disease implies a weakness, trouble, failure that is mechanical; there is no disgrace, nothing of the taboo that once surrounded people afflicted with TB and still surrounds those who have cancer' (Sontag, p. 12).

TB?
Cancer? –'The dying tubercular is pictured as made more beautiful and more soulful; the person dying of cancer is portrayed as
robbed of all capacity of self-transcendence, humiliated by fear
and agony' (Sontag, p. 20).
AIDS?

Are certain diseases fashionable?

Do our preoccupations with certain diseases follow fashions?
Is health fashionable, as fashionable as it could be (as fashionable
as stress)?
Is a healthy image a positive one (to whom)?

**What are the implications of these issues – and of our answers
to these questions – for the education of carers?**

Sontag's text, therefore, revealed, or prompted debate on, how we represent illness. It is not just a matter of the words we choose to use –
although these can be revealing too – it is a matter of how we concep-
tualize and fantasize about illness, whether or not we are actually ill or
dealing with people who are. This discussion made us much more
conscious, for a while, of our own and each other's choice of words.
Above all, Sontag's text again takes us away from strictly medical writing; this is more like the 'sociology' of medicine, but each reader could
use it to interrogate some of their own assumptions about these illnesses and perhaps some of their own assumptions about other people's views of these illnesses.

This is another variation on the theme of scientific subject meeting
non-scientific approach and style of writing. It is non-scientific in the
sense that it does not adhere to the conventions of medical writing; it
is, however, scientific in its use of logic, argument and sources.

In medical humanities we have frequently explored imagery and
metaphors for illness and thereby gained insights into different views
of illnesses, often the patient's point of view. Sontag has prompted us
to move beyond this acceptance of metaphor as a revelation of point
of view. She has made us consider the process of making metaphors:

> **Why do we use them?**
>
> **When do we use them?**
>
> Is it because we do not want to use medical language?
> Is it because we do not know the medical terms well enough to know how to use them?
> Is it because no-one else uses the medical terms?
> Is it because we fear that other people may not be comfortable with them?
> Is it because medical people have helped us to find metaphors for a condition, thinking that this will make it easier for us to understand or cope?
> Is it because we want to help other people to understand or cope?

Are metaphors, therefore, distancing devices, creating a space between us and the reality of illness? Or do they help us to express our experience or our awareness of them?

The final text in this chapter could serve as an illustration of the approach Sontag is looking for. In *Able Lives: Women's Experience of Paralysis*, the first-hand accounts of injuries and treatments are descriptive rather than metaphorical. These are narrative accounts of experiences rather than creative writings. For example, one of the women describes how she managed her return to a way of life quite close to what she had known before her accident:

Bridget's consultant told her, 'I would be quite capable of returning home to look after my 13-month-old daughter ... until, that is, he found out that I was a single parent living on my own. I was, of course, able to look after my daughter without any help at all, but only because the local authority provided me with a flat which was suitable for someone in a wheelchair. I was then able to return to work and carry on life as a single working mother, but again only because there were certain physical things that made this possible – the building in which I worked was accessible; I could drive and could afford the deposit for a car leased through Motability; the local authority subsidized the cost of a childminder and also provided me with a home help to do my housework. All these things facilitated my return to life as it was before my accident; without them I couldn't have done it'. This again emphasizes the lack of physical and material resources as major problems, and it is these things which handicap us, not our disabilities. p. 129

This description usefully adjusts perceptions of this woman's position – and each of the women included in this book describes her life differently. One thing many of them have in common is pain, and I used their writings on this subject with a group of third-year under-graduate Prosthetics and Orthotics students to prompt discussion of their role in helping patients come to terms with and manage pain. Extracts from this text that dealt with the subject of pain triggered an interesting discussion in which the students disagreed with each other on the question of whether or not it was 'right' for these women to use alcohol and smoking for pain management.

Many aspects of these women's experiences are described by the women themselves, including their emotional responses to the injury and to their carers. While many carers would be concerned to help these women make the adjustment to their new lives, one of the women said that she would have appreciated more help to 'plan our future'. In help-ing people cope with illness, do we give them enough help to visualize, fantasize and realize a future? Do we help **them** to 'move on'?

The readings in this chapter have been selected to show the wide range of texts about scientific and medical subjects in a wide range of styles. Each of these texts tackles its subject in a different way and it would be difficult to generalize across these readings about a 'new style of scientific or medical writing'.

Each way of writing brings with it a particular way of 'knowing' the subject, a different way of accounting for experience, even, in some examples, a different way of recording observations. In fact, some of these texts have argued that no one way of knowing is adequate; we need to look at situations and people from different angles if we are truly to understand their condition and genuinely to communicate with them.

So, the distinction between scientific and non-scientific, between medical and non-medical, between 'facts' and imaginings has come to seem an oversimplification. Although it has often happened, one should not displace the other.

In the context of the health professions, in particular, perhaps this distinction could prevent us from genuinely caring, caring for the whole person and not just caring for the condition. Perhaps medical humanities can help us to see the patient 'in the round', i.e. not only from more than one point of view but also in more than one way, as revealed in our ability to use more than one 'set of words'.

Perhaps medical humanities is an emerging model of reflective practice; without a mechanism for reflection how does it develop? Even if reflection is to happen in practice, when do we develop the skills and confidence to reflect in this way?

Medical humanities is one way of bringing together theory and practice, in writing and talking and taking time to look at ways in which we can 'move on' from our own patterns of practice.

Moreover, medical humanities can help us to avoid the territorialism that keeps different disciplines separate in different departments and domains; it can create a forum where the disciplines can learn to talk to each other. If nothing else, medical humanities can give us time to think about the 'territory' we inhabit, about whether or not we are comfortable in it and how we might be able to move away from it. Perhaps our medical humanities group has established a new territory? As an autonomous group, we are engaging in fewer, if any, territorial battles. We have no budget to defend, for example. While this is a pleasant relief, perhaps we will find that we have to defend this territory.

But this is only my view; I wonder what kind of book other participants in our group would, or will, write. Simply being in the group has given me confidence to develop my ideas in this book. The writing practice has got me into the writing 'habit'.

So, what is it all about? Medical humanities is **not** about making us all literary scholars. It is **not** about making us all better carers. It **is** about facing up to different views, about learning to deal with ambiguity, and about beginning to deal with difficult issues. It is also stimulating, unpredictable and – we must not forget – fun.

The last word must be autonomous: if it is an autonomous group, you can make it whatever you like.

Bibliography

Literary texts

Barrington, J. (ed.) (1991) *An Intimate Wilderness: Lesbian Writers on Sexuality*, Eighth Mountain, Portland, OR.

Brown, G. M. (1976) *Winterfold*, Hogarth Press, London.

Burns, R. (1969) *Poems and Songs*, (ed. J. Kinsley), Oxford University Press, Oxford.

Butler, S. (1991) Cancer in two voices: living in my changing body, in *An Intimate Wilderness: Lesbian Writers on Sexuality*, (ed. J. Barrington), Eighth Mountain, Portland, OR, pp. 139–143.

Crichton, M. (1991) *Jurassic Park*, Arrow Books, London.

Dunn, D. (1985) *Elegies*, Faber, London.

Fraser, C. M. (1980) *Blue Above the Chimneys*, Fontana, Glasgow.

Galloway, J. (1992) *The Trick is to Keep Breathing*, Minerva, London.

Jennings, E. (1987) *Collected Poems, 1953–86*, Carcanet, Manchester.

Kydd, R. (1987) *Auld Zimmery*, Mariscat, Glasgow.

Lapierre, D. (1986) *City of Joy*, Arrow Books, London.

McWilliam, C. (1989) *A Little Stranger*, Picador, London.

Murphy, R. F. (1990) *The Body Silent*, Norton, London.

Rich, A. (1984) *The Fact of a Doorframe, Poems Selected and New, 1950–1984*, Norton, London.

Rosenblum, B. (1991) Cancer in two voices: living in an unstable body, in *An Intimate Wilderness: Lesbian Writers on Sexuality*, (ed. J. Barrington), Eighth Mountain, Portland, OR, pp. 133–138.

Sergeant, H. (1980) *Poems from the Medical World*, MTP Press, Lancaster.

Whitaker, A. (ed.) (1992) *All in the End is Harvest: An Anthology for Those Who Grieve*, Longman & Todd, London.

Non-literary texts

Bolton, G. (1994) Stories at work. Fictional–critical writing as a means of professional development. *British Educational Research Journal*, **20**(1), 55–68.

Bouchard, C., Shephard, R. J. and Stephens, T. (eds) (1994) *Physical Activity, Fitness, and Health: International Consensus Statement*, Human Kinetics, Windsor, Ontario.

Burnard, P. (1992) *Effective Communication Skills for Health Professionals*, Chapman & Hall, London.

Calman, K. C. and Downie, R. S. (1988) Education and training in medicine. *Medical Education*, **22**, 488–491.

Casement, P. (1990) *Further Learning from the Patient*, Routledge, London.

Christensen, C. R. *et al.* (eds) (1991) *Education for Judgement: The Artistry of Discussion Leadership*, Harvard Business School, Boston, MA.

Clawsen, A. L. (1994) The relationship between clinical decision making and ethical decision making. *Physiotherapy*, **80**(1), 10–14.

Collier, J. (1989) Medical education as abuse. *British Medical Journal*, **299**, 1408–1409.

Dias, W. P. S. (1995) Reflective practice in engineering design. *Civil Engineering*, **108**, 160–168.

Elbow, P. (1973) *Writing Without Teachers*, Oxford University Press, Oxford.

Elbow, P. (1981) *Writing with Power: Techniques for Mastering the Writing Process*, Oxford University Press, Oxford.

Fallowfield, L. (1990) *The Quality of Life: The Missing Measurement in Health Care*, Souvenir Press, London.

Gaba, M. (1991) The right treatment for visiting people in hospital. *The Herald* (Glasgow), **5 February**, p. 10.

Gersie, A. and King, N. (1990) *Storymaking in Education and Therapy*, Jessica Kingsley, London.

Gleick, J. (1987) *Chaos, Making a New Science*, Abacus, London.

Grasha, T. (1990) Practical poetry: using metaphors to evaluate academic programs. *Journal of Staff, Program, and Organization Development*, **8**(1), 23–32.

Gribbin, J. (1984) *In Search of Schrödinger's Cat*, Corgi, London.

Ley, P. (1988) *Communicating with Patients*, Chapman & Hall, London.

Lowrie, S. (1992) Medical education: what's wrong with medical education in Britain? *British Medical Journal*, **305**, 1277–1280.

Lowrie, S. (1992) Medical education: student selection. *British Medical Journal*, **305**, 1352–1354.

Lowrie, S. (1992) Medical education: strategies for implementing curriculum change. *British Medical Journal*, **305**, 1482–1485.

Lowrie, S. (1993) Medical education: assessment of students. *British Medical Journal*, **306**, 51–54.

Lowrie, S. (1993) Medical education: teaching the teachers. *British Medical Journal*, **306**, 127–130.

Lowrie, S. (1993) Medical education: the preregistration year. *British Medical Journal*, **306**, 196–198.

Lowrie, S. (1993) Medical education: trends in health care and their effects on medical education. *British Medical Journal*, **306**, 255–258.

Lowrie, S. (1993) Medical education: making change happen. *British Medical Journal*, **306**, 320–322.

Macdonald, C. (1992) *Could it be Stress?: Reflections on Psychosomatic Illness*, Argyll, Glendaruel.

May, W. F. (1985) The virtues and vices of the elderly. *Socio-Economic Planning Sciences*, **19**(4), 255–262.

Medawar, P. (1984) *The Limits of Science*, Oxford University Press, Oxford.

Morris, J. (1993) An overview of and comparison among three current approaches to medical and physiotherapy undergraduate education. *Physiotherapy*, **79**(2), 91–94.

Morris, J. (ed.) (1989) *Able Lives: Women's Experience of Paralysis*, Women's Press, London.

Newton, R. and Wilkinson, M. J. (1994) When the talking is over: using action learning. *Management Development Review*, **7**(2), 9–15.

Paffenbarger, R. S. *et al.* (1994) Some interrelations of physical activity, physiological fitness, health, and longevity, in *Physical Activity, Fitness, and Health: International Proceedings and Consensus Statement*, (eds C. Bouchard *et al.*), Human Kinetics, Windsor, ON, pp. 119–133.

Sachs, O. (1990) *Awakenings*, Picador, London.

Sarton, M. (1988) *After the Stroke: A Journal*, Women's Press, London.

Schon, D. A. (1987) *Educating the Reflective Practitioner: Towards a New Design for Teaching and Learning in the Professions*, Jossey-Bass, San Francisco, CA.

Sim, J. (1990) The concept of health. *Physiotherapy*, **76**(7), 423–428.

Simpson, M. *et al.* (1991) Doctor–patient communication: the Toronto consensus statement. *British Medical Journal*, **303**, 1385–1387.

Sontag, S. (1977) *Illness as Metaphor*, Penguin, Harmondsworth.

Wheelan, G. (1988) Improving medical students' clinical problem-solving, in *Improving Learning: New Perspectives*, (ed. P. Ramsden), Kogan Page, London.

White, M. and Epstein, D. (1990) *Narrative Means to Therapeutic Ends*, Norton, New York.

Medical humanities

Breo, D. L. (1990) M. Therese Southgate, MD – the woman behind 'The Cover'. *Journal of the American Medical Association*, **263**(15), 2107–2112.

Calman, K. C. *et al.* (1988) Literature and medicine: a short course for medical students. *Medical Education*, **22**, 265–269.

Charon, R. *et al.* (1995) Literature and medicine: contributions to clinical practice. *Annals of Internal Medicine*, **122**, 599–606.

Bibliography

Darbyshire, P. (1994) Understanding caring through arts and humanities: a medical/nursing humanities approach to promoting alternative experiences of thinking and learning. *Journal of Advanced Nursing*, **19**, 850–863.

Murray, R. (1994) Medical humanities: a practical introduction. *Physiotherapy Ireland*, **15**(1), 25–29.

Murray, R. and Thow, M. (1995) A medical humanities roadshow: 'spreading the word'. *Physiotherapy*, **81**(2), 95–106.

Radwany, S. M. and Adelson, B. H. (1987) The use of literary classics in teaching medical ethics to physicians. *Journal of the American Medical Association*, **257** (12), 1629–1631.

Robb, A. and Murray, R. (1992) Medical Humanities in nursing: thought provoking? *Journal of Advanced Nursing*, **17**, 1182–1187.

Rogers, J. (1994) Doubts about medical humanities. *Health Care Analysis*, **2**, 347–350.

Self, D. J. (1993) The educational philosophies behind the Medical Humanities programs in the United States: an empirical assessment of three different approaches to humanistic medical education. *Theoretical Medicine*, **14**, 221–229.

Thow, M. and Murray, R. (1991) Medical humanities in physiotherapy: education and practice. *Physiotherapy*, **77**(11), 733–736.

Warren, K. S. (1984) The humanities in medical education. *Annals of Internal Medicine*, **101**, 697–701.

Wear, D. W. (1992) The colonization of medical humanities: a confessional critique. *Journal of Medical Humanities*, **13**(4), 199–209.

Young-Mason, J. (1988) Literature as a mirror to compassion. *Journal of Professional Nursing*, **4**(4), 299–301.

Index